The Bethesda System for Reporting
Thyroid Cytopathology

Syed Z. Ali • Edmund S. Cibas
Editors

The Bethesda System for Reporting Thyroid Cytopathology

Definitions, Criteria and Explanatory Notes

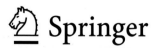 Springer

Editors
Syed Z. Ali, MD
The Johns Hopkins Hospital
Baltimore, MD
USA
sali@jhmi.edu

Edmund S. Cibas, MD
Harvard Medical School
Brigham and Women's Hospital
Boston, MA
USA
ecibas@partners.org

ISBN 978-0-387-87665-8   e-ISBN 978-0-387-87666-5
DOI 10.1007/978-0-387-87666-5
Springer New York Dordrecht Heidelberg London

Library of Congress Control Number: 2009932423

Printed on acid-free paper

Springer is part of Springer Science+Business Media (www.springer.com)

Preface

This atlas is the offspring of the "The National Cancer Institute (NCI) Thyroid Fine Needle Aspiration (FNA) State of the Science Conference," hosted by the NCI and organized by Dr. Andrea Abati. Preparations for the conference began 18 months earlier with the designation of a steering committee and the establishment of a dedicated, permanent web site. The meeting took place on October 22 and 23, 2007 in Bethesda, Maryland and was co-moderated by Susan J. Mandel and Edmund S. Cibas.

The discussions and conclusions regarding terminology and morphologic criteria from the meeting were summarized in publications by Baloch et al.[1, 2] and form the framework for this atlas. The atlas is organized by the general categories of "Nondiagnostic," "Benign," "Follicular Neoplasm/Suspicious for a Follicular Neoplasm", "Suspicious for Malignancy," and "Malignant," and it includes the definitions and morphologic criteria of these categories as set forth by Baloch et al. The majority of the conference participants also agreed on a category of "undetermined significance," which is incorporated in this atlas (Chap. 4).

It is critical that the cytopathologist communicate thyroid FNA interpretations to the referring physician in terms that are succinct, unambiguous, and helpful clinically. We recognize that the terminology used here is a flexible framework that can be modified by individual laboratories to meet the needs of their providers and the patients they serve. Historically, terminology for thyroid FNA has varied markedly from one laboratory to another, creating confusion in some instances and hindering the sharing of data among multiple institutions. It is the hope of all the contributors to this atlas that it will be a valuable supplement to the Terminology committee's extraodinary summary document.

Syed Z. Ali   Edmund S. Cibas

References

1. Baloch ZW, Cibas ES, Clark DP, Layfield LJ, Ljung BM, Pitman MB, et al. The National Cancer Institute Thyroid fine needle aspiration state of the science conference: a summation. Cytojournal 2008;5:6.
2. Baloch ZW, LiVolsi VA, Asa SL, Rosai J, Merino MJ, Randolph G, et al. Diagnostic terminology and morphologic criteria for cytologic diagnosis of thyroid lesions: a synopsis of the National Cancer Institute Thyroid Fine-Needle Aspiration State of the Science Conference. Diagn Cytopathol 2008;36(6):425–37.

Contents

Contributors

Pedro Patricio de Agustin, M.D., Ph.D.
Department of Pathology, University Hospital "12 de Octubre," Madrid, Spain

Erik K. Alexander, M.D.
Department of Medicine, Brigham and Women's Hospital and Harvard Medical School, Boston, MA, USA

Sylvia L. Asa, M.D., Ph.D.
Department of Pathology and Laboratory Medicine, University of Toronto; University Health Network and Toronto Medical Laboratories; Ontario Cancer Institute, Toronto, ON, Canada

Kristen A. Atkins, M.D.
Department of Pathology, University of Virginia Health System, Charlottesville, VA, USA

Manon Auger, M.D.
Department of Pathology, McGill University Health Center and McGill University, Montreal, QC, Canada

Zubair W. Baloch, M.D., Ph.D.
Department of Pathology and Laboratory Medicine, University of Pennsylvania Medical Center, Philadelphia, PA, USA

Katherine Berezowski, M.D.
Department of Pathology, Virginia Hospital Center, Arlington, VA, USA

Massimo Bongiovanni, M.D.
Department of Pathology, Geneva University Hospital, Geneva, Switzerland

Douglas P. Clark, M.D.
Department of Pathology, The Johns Hopkins Medical Institutions, Baltimore, MD, USA

Béatrix Cochand-Priollet, M.D., Ph.D.
Department of Pathology, Lariboisière Hospital, University of Paris 7, Paris, France

Barbara A. Crothers, D.O.
Department of Pathology, Walter Reed Army Medical Center, Springfield, VA, USA

Richard M. DeMay, M.D.
Department of Pathology, University of Chicago, Chicago, IL, USA

Tarik M. Elsheikh, M.D.
Ball Memorial Hospital/PA Labs, Muncie, IN, USA

William C. Faquin, M.D., Ph.D.
Department of Pathology, Massachusetts General Hospital and Harvard Medical School, Boston, MA, USA

Armando C. Filie, M.D.
Laboratory of Pathology, National Cancer Institute, Bethesda, MD, USA

Pinar Firat, M.D.
Department of Pathology, Hacettepe University, Ankara, Turkey

William J. Frable, M.D.
Department of Pathology, Medical College of Virginia Hospitals, Virginia Commonwealth University Medical Center, Richmond, VA, USA

Kim R. Geisinger, M.D.
Department of Pathology, Wake Forest University School of Medicine, Winston-Salem, NC, USA

Hossein Gharib, M.D.
Department of Endocrinology, Mayo Clinic College of Medicine, Rochester, MN, USA

Ulrike M. Hamper, M.D.
Department of Radiology and Radiological Sciences, The Johns Hopkins Medical Institutions, Baltimore, MD, USA

Michael R. Henry, M.D.
Department of Laboratory Medicine and Pathology, Mayo Clinic and Foundation, Rochester, MN, USA

Jeffrey F. Krane, M.D, Ph.D.
Department of Pathology, Brigham and Women's Hospital and Harvard Medical School, Boston, MA, USA

Lester J. Layfield, M.D.
Department of Pathology, University of Utah Hospital and Clinics, Salt Lake City, UT, USA

Virginia A. LiVolsi, M.D.
Departments of Pathology and Laboratory Medicine, University of Pennsylvania Medical Center, Philadelphia, PA, USA

Britt-Marie E. Ljung, M.D.
Departments of Pathology and Laboratory Medicine, University of California San Francisco, San Francisco, CA, USA

Claire W. Michael, M.D.
Department of Pathology, University of Michigan Medical Center, Ann Arbor, MI, USA

Ritu Nayar, M.D.
Department of Pathology, Northwestern University, Feinberg School of Medicine, Chicago, IL, USA

Yolanda C. Oertel, M.D.
Department of Pathology, Washington Hospital Center, Washington, DC, USA

Martha B. Pitman, M.D.
Department of Pathology, Massachusetts General Hospital and Harvard Medical School, Boston, MA, USA

Celeste N. Powers, M.D., Ph.D.
Department of Pathology, Medical College of Virginia Hospitals, Virginia Commonwealth University Medical Center, Richmond, VA, USA

Stephen S. Raab, M.D.
Department of Pathology, University of Colorado at Denver, UCDHSC Anschutz Medical Campus, Aurora, CO, USA

Andrew A. Renshaw, M.D.
Department of Pathology, Baptist Hospital of Miami, Miami, FL, USA

Juan Rosai, M.D.
Dipartimento di Patologia, Instituto Nazionale Tumori, Milano, Italy

Miguel A. Sanchez, M.D.
Department of Pathology, Englewood Hospital and Medical Center, Englewood, NJ, USA

Vinod Shidham, M.D.
Department of Pathology, Medical College of Wisconsin, Milwaukee, WI, USA

Mary K. Sidawy, M.D.
Department of Pathology, Georgetown University Medical Center, Washington, DC, USA

Gregg A. Staerkel, M.D.
Department of Pathology, The University of Texas M.D. Anderson Cancer Center, Houston, TX, USA

Edward B. Stelow, M.D.
Department of Pathology, University of Virginia Health System, Charlottesville, VA, USA

Jerry Waisman, M.D.
Department of Pathology, New York University of Medicine, New York, NY, USA

Helen H. Wang, M.D., Dr.P.H.
Department of Pathology, Beth Israel Deaconess Medical Center and Harvard Medical School, Boston, MA, USA

Philippe Vielh, M.D., Ph.D.
Department of Pathology, Institut de Cancerologie Gustave Roussy, Villejuif, France

Grace C. H. Yang, M.D.
Department of Pathology, Weill Medical College of Cornell University, New York, NY, USA

Matthew A. Zarka, M.D.
Department of Laboratory Medicine and Pathology, Mayo Clinic Arizona, Scottsdale, AZ, USA

Abbreviations

AUS	Atypia of undetermined significance
BFN	Benign follicular nodule
BSRTC	Bethesda System for Reporting Thyroid Cytopathology
FLUS	Follicular lesion of undetermined significance
FMTC	Familial medullary thyroid carcinoma
FN	Follicular neoplasm
FNA	Fine needle aspiration
FNHCT	Follicular neoplasm, Hürthle cell type
FVPTC	Follicular variant of papillary thyroid carcinoma
GD	Graves' disease
HCN	Hürthle cell neoplasm
HTT	Hyalinizing trabecular tumor
INCI	Intranuclear cytoplasmic pseudoinclusion
LBP	Liquid-based preparations
LT	Lymphocytic thyroiditis
MALT	Mucosa-associated lymphoid tissue
MEN	Multiple endocrine neoplasia
MM	Malignant melanoma
MNG	Multinodular goiter
MTC	Medullary thyroid carcinoma
N/C	Nuclear/cytoplasmic
NCI	National Cancer Institute, Bethesda, MD
NG	Nodular goiter
NSE	Neuron specific enolase
PB	Psammoma body
PDTC	Poorly differentiated thyroid carcinoma
PPV	Positive predictive value
PTC	Papillary thyroid carcinoma

PTH	Parathyroid hormone
RCC	Renal cell carcinoma
SFM	Suspicious for malignancy
SFN	Suspicious for a follicular neoplasm
SFNHCT	Suspicious for a follicular neoplasm, Hürthle cell type
SmCC	Small cell carcinoma
SQC	Squamous cell carcinoma
TCV	Tall cell variant
UTC	Undifferentiated (anaplastic) carcinoma
WHO	World Health Organization

Chapter 1

Overview of Diagnostic Terminology and Reporting

Zubair W. Baloch, Erik K. Alexander,
Hossein Gharib, and Stephen S. Raab

Fine needle aspiration (FNA) plays an essential role in the evaluation of the euthyroid patient with a thyroid nodule: it reduces unnecessary surgery for patients with benign nodules and appropriately triages patients with malignant nodules for timely clinical intervention. It is critical, therefore, that the cytopathologist communicate thyroid FNA interpretations to the referring physician in terms that are succinct, unambiguous, and clinically useful.

Format of the Report

For clarity of communication, the Bethesda System for Reporting Thyroid Cytopathology (BSRTC) recommends that each thyroid FNA report begin with a general diagnostic category. The BSRTC diagnostic categories are shown in Table 1.1. Each category has an implied cancer risk, which ranges from 0% to 3% for the "Benign" category to virtually 100% for the "Malignant" category. As a function of these risk associations, each category is linked to evidence-based clinical management guidelines, as shown in Table 1.2 and discussed in more detail in the chapters that follow.

For several categories, a consensus on a single name was not reached at the NCI Conference (Table 1.1); either term is considered acceptable.

For some of the general categories, some degree of subcategorization can be informative and is often appropriate; recommended terminology is shown in Table 1.1. Additional descriptive comments (beyond such subcategorization) are optional and left to the discretion of the cytopathologist.

Notes and recommendations are not required but can be useful in certain circumstances. Some laboratories, for example, may wish to state the risk

Syed Z. Ali and Edmund S. Cibas (eds.), *The Bethesda System for Reporting
Thyroid Cytopathology*, DOI 10.1007/ 978-0-387-87666-5_1,
© Springer Science+Business Media, LLC 2010

TABLE 1.1. The Bethesda System for Reporting Thyroid Cytopathology; recommended diagnostic categories.

I. Nondiagnostic or Unsatisfactory
Cyst fluid only
Virtually acellular specimen
Other (obscuring blood, clotting artifact, etc.)

II. Benign
Consistent with a benign follicular nodule (includes adenomatoid nodule, colloid nodule, etc.)
Consistent with lymphocytic (Hashimoto) thyroiditis in the proper clinical context
Consistent with granulomatous (subacute) thyroiditis
Other

III. Atypia of Undetermined Significance or Follicular Lesion of Undetermined Significance

IV. Follicular Neoplasm or Suspicious for a Follicular Neoplasm
specify if Hürthle cell (oncocytic) type

V. Suspicious for Malignancy
Suspicious for papillary carcinoma
Suspicious for medullary carcinoma
Suspicious for metastatic carcinoma
Suspicious for lymphoma
Other

VI. Malignant
Papillary thyroid carcinoma
Poorly differentiated carcinoma
Medullary thyroid carcinoma
Undifferentiated (anaplastic) carcinoma
Squamous cell carcinoma
Carcinoma with mixed features (specify)
Metastatic carcinoma
Non-Hodgkin lymphoma
Other

of malignancy associated with the general category, based on its own cytologic–histologic correlation or that found in the literature (Table 1.2). Sample reports, which we hope will be a useful guide, are provided in the remaining chapters.

TABLE **1.2.** The Bethesda system for reporting thyroid cytopathology: implied risk of malignancy and recommended clinical management.

Diagnostic category	Risk of malignancy(%)	Usual management[a]
Nondiagnostic or Unsatisfactory	[b]	Repeat FNA with ultrasound guidance
Benign	0–3	Clinical follow-up
Atypia of Undetermined Significance or Follicular Lesion of Undetermined Significance	~5–15[c]	Repeat FNA
Follicular Neoplasm or Suspicious for a Follicular Neoplasm	15–30	Surgical lobectomy
Suspicious for Malignancy	60–75	Near-total thyroidectomy or surgical lobectomy[d]
Malignant	97–99	Near-total thyroidectomy[d]

[a]Actual management may depend on other factors (e.g., clinical, sonographic) besides the FNA interpretation

[b]See Chap. 2 for discussion

[c]Estimate extrapolated from histopathologic data from patients with "repeated atypicals" (Yang J et al. Fine-Needle Aspiration of Thyroid Nodules: A Study of 4703 Patients with Histologic and Clinical Correlations. *Cancer* 2007;111: 306–15; Yassa L et al. Long-Term Assessment of a Multi-disciplinary Approach to Thyroid Nodule Diagnostic Evaluation. *Cancer* 2007;111: 508–16.)

[d]In the case of "Suspicious for metastatic tumor" or a "Malignant" interpretation indicating metastatic tumor rather than a primary thyroid malignancy, surgery may not be indicated

Chapter 2

Nondiagnostic/Unsatisfactory

Barbara A. Crothers, Michael R. Henry,
Pinar Firat, and Ulrike M. Hamper

Background

In order to provide useful diagnostic information for optimal clinical management, a fine needle aspiration (FNA) sample of a thyroid nodule should be representative of the underlying lesion. A good criterion of adequacy, when appropriately applied, ensures a low false-negative rate. It is worth emphasizing, however, that cellularity/adequacy is dependent not only on the technique of the aspirator, but also on the inherent nature of the lesion (e.g., solid *vs.* cystic). In general, the adequacy of a thyroid FNA is defined by both the quantity and quality of the cellular and colloid components.

An assessment of specimen adequacy is an integral component of an FNA interpretation because it conveys the degree of certainty with which one can rely on the result. The definition of an adequate specimen in thyroid FNA is subjective and controversial. While the *quality* of a specimen is irrefutably critical to proper interpretation, controversy is introduced when rigid numerical criteria for cell *quantity* are imposed. No study supports any specific follicular cellularity as applicable to all cases (benign and malignant, cystic and solid) with high diagnostic accuracy. Additionally, there is no consensus supporting a minimum number of FNA passes required to obtain adequate samples. High quality specimens contain sufficient cells representative of a lesion to allow the observer to confidently render an accurate interpretation. High quality requires proficient collection combined with excellent slide preparation, processing, and staining.

Historically, the terms "nondiagnostic" and "inadequate/unsatisfactory" have been used interchangeably by some but not all cytopathologists: some cytopathologists (and endocrinologists) have interpreted the terms to mean different things.[1] An unsatisfactory specimen is always nondiagnostic, but some technically satisfactory specimens may also be considered "nondiagnostic," that is, showing nonspecific features not conclusively diagnostic of a particular entity. At the NCI conference, the terms "Nondiagnostic (ND)" and "Unsatisfactory (UNS)" were recommended for the category that conveys an inadequate/insufficient sample.[2] The Bethesda System is a flexible framework, however, and can be modified by the laboratory to suit the needs of its providers. Thus, if neither ND nor UNS appeals to providers, a more descriptive term like "Insufficient for Diagnosis" can be substituted. For the sake of simplicity, however, ND is used throughout the atlas to convey a sample that does not meet the adequacy criteria outlined below.

Definition

A specimen is considered "Nondiagnostic" or "Unsatisfactory" if it fails to meet the following adequacy criteria.

Criteria for Adequacy

A thyroid FNA sample is considered adequate for evaluation if it contains a minimum of six groups of well-visualized (i.e., well-stained, undistorted, and unobstructed) follicular cells, with at least ten cells per group, preferably on a single slide. Exceptions to this requirement apply to the following special circumstances:

1. *Solid nodules with cytologic atypia.* A sample that contains significant cytologic atypia is never considered ND/UNS. It is mandatory to report any significant atypia; a minimum number of follicular cells is not required.
2. *Solid nodules with inflammation.* Nodules in patients with lymphocytic (Hashimoto) thyroiditis, thyroid abscess, or granulomatous thyroiditis may contain only numerous inflammatory cells. Such cases are interpreted as Benign and not as ND/UNS. A minimum number of follicular cells is not required.
3. *Colloid nodules.* Specimens that consist of abundant thick colloid are considered Benign and satisfactory for evaluation. A minimum number of follicular cells is not required if easily-identifiable colloid predominates.

Nondiagnostic/Unsatisfactory (Figs. 2.1–2.7)

The following scenarios describe cases considered Nondiagnostic:

1. Fewer than six groups of well-preserved, well-stained follicular cell groups with ten cells each (see exceptions above)
2. Poorly prepared, poorly stained, or obscured follicular cells
3. Cyst fluid, with or without histiocytes, and fewer than six groups of ten benign follicular cells (see Explanatory Notes)

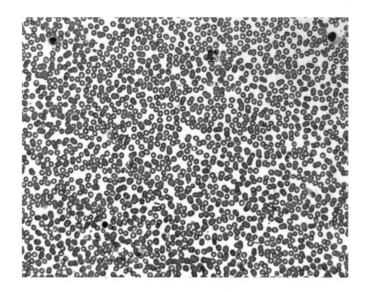

FIGURE 2.1. Nondiagnostic. The smear shows abundant red cells, with rare lymphocytes and monocytes. The sample is devoid of thyroid parenchymal elements. Some thyroid nodules are very vascular and on repeated passes yield only blood. Employing a smaller gauge needle (27 gauge), avoiding negative pressure, and employing a shorter needle dwell time within the nodule often results in better cellularity (smear, Diff-Quik stain).

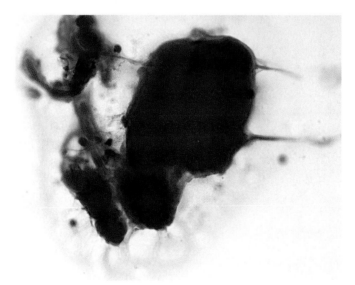

FIGURE 2.2. Nondiagnostic. The smear shows a large fragment of skeletal muscle and no native thyroid tissue. This may occur when the needle traverses through the neck muscles. It is important not to confuse skeletal muscle with inspissated colloid (notice the cross striations in the muscle fragment, best seen at 7 o'clock) (smear, Papanicolaou stain).

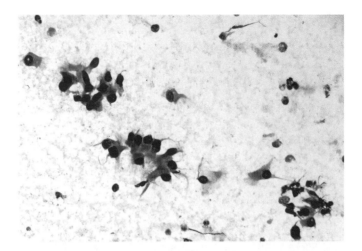

FIGURE 2.3. Nondiagnostic. This FNA yielded ciliated respiratory epithelium from the trachea. Accidental puncture of the tracheal lumen is uncommon and typically happens in lesions of the thyroid isthmus. Such cases should be carefully evaluated for adequacy since they typically show only rare follicular epithelium (smear, Diff-Quik stain).

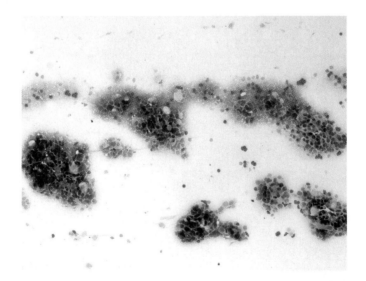

FIGURE 2.4. Nondiagnostic. Extensive air-drying artifact in this alcohol-fixed smear makes the cytologic interpretation difficult. Such cases should be carefully evaluated for adequacy and are best managed by a repeat FNA with rapid wet-fixation. Liquid-based cytology often resolves such issues and may be considered if air-drying artifact is a repeated problem (smear, Papanicolaou stain).

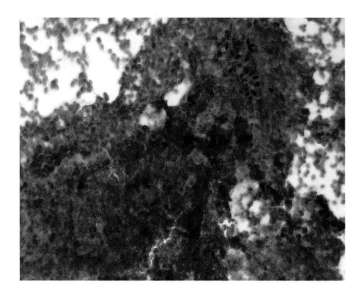

Figure 2.5. Nondiagnostic. Extensive obscuring blood hinders the evaluation of the follicular cells (smear, Papanicolaou stain).

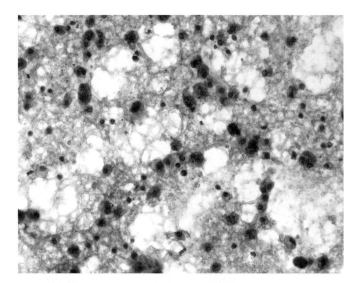

Figure 2.6. Nondiagnostic (cyst fluid only). Abundant hemosiderin-laden macrophages and degenerated cyst fluid contents. Macrophages do not count towards specimen adequacy. Such cases, when devoid of significant background colloid, are interpreted as Nondiagnostic (smear, Papanicolaou stain).

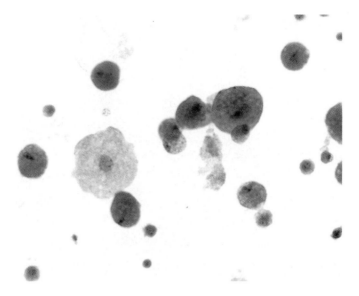

Figure 2.7. Nondiagnostic (cyst fluid only). Macrophages are typically noncohesive, with abundant cytoplasm which often contains golden-brown hemosiderin pigment with the Papanicolaou stain (SurePath preparation, Papanicolaou stain; case courtesy of Douglas R. Schneider, MD, Excell Clinical Laboratories, Boston, MA, USA).

Explanatory Notes

Adequate samples are required to prevent false negative reports of thyroid lesions.[3] Recommendations for adequacy generally apply only to the quantity of follicular cells and exclude consideration of macrophages, lymphocytes, and other nonmalignant cellular components.[4,5] The ability to obtain follicular cells by FNA is dependent, in part, upon the nature of the lesion. The number of follicular cells necessary for a diagnosis is contingent upon the lesion aspirated because some lesions, such as benign cysts, do not yield many follicular cells.

Solid nodules with cytologic atypia should always be considered adequate and reported as abnormal ("Atypia of Undetermined Significance," "Suspicious for Malignancy," etc., depending on the findings), with a comment describing any limiting factor(s) such as scant cellularity. Follicular cells are not always present in aspirates of inflammatory lesions such as lymphocytic thyroiditis, thyroid abscesses, or granulomatous thyroiditis. Therefore, there is no minimum requirement for a follicular component when inflammation predominates. The presence of abundant colloid (as opposed to serum; Figs. 2.8 and 2.9) reliably identifies most benign processes

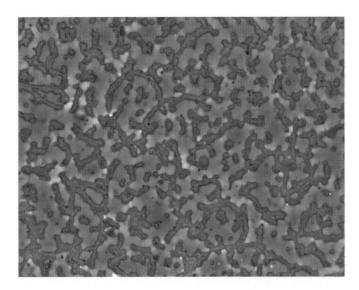

FIGURE 2.8. Benign (satisfactory thyroid FNA). Abundant colloid coats the smear in this case of a "colloid nodule." Aspirates with large amounts of colloid are considered adequate for interpretation even when they contain less the six groups of follicular cells (smear, Diff-Quik stain).

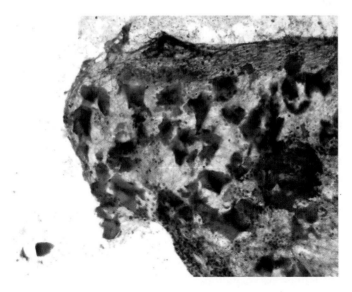

FIGURE 2.9. Benign (satisfactory thyroid FNA). There is abundant dense colloid but only scant follicular cells (smear, Papanicolaou stain).

despite scant follicular cells.[6] One group of follicular cells with features sufficient for the diagnosis of papillary thyroid carcinoma may constitute an adequate specimen in the proper clinical setting and should not be considered Nondiagnostic despite scant cellularity.[7]

Cyst fluid may yield only macrophages, but the risk of malignancy is low for these lesions if they are simple and under 3 cm.[4,8,9] The cytopathologist is not always privy to clinical/sonographic information, however, and, in isolation, the possibility of a cystic papillary thyroid carcinoma cannot be excluded if a sample consists almost entirely of fluid and histiocytes. For this reason, such cases are reported as ND/UNS followed by the subcategory "Cyst fluid only" (See Sample Report 2). In the proper clinical setting (e.g., ultrasound evidence of a simple, unilocular cyst), these specimens may be considered clinically adequate, even though they are reported as ND/UNS.[4]

Occasionally, an adjacent anatomic site is aspirated, such as the trachea (Fig. 2.3) or sternocleidomastoid muscle (Fig. 2.2), yielding only nonthyroidal tissue. Such cases are considered ND/UNS.

There does not appear to be any difference in specimen adequacy using follicular cells in liquid-based preparations (LBP) as opposed to conventional smears. A minimum number of cell clusters is not as important as the total number of follicular cells in LBP, with 180–320 providing a diagnostic agreement of 80%.[10]

In the Bethesda System, unless a sample is interpreted as ND/UNS, it is considered satisfactory for evaluation.

Management

Nodules with an initial ND/UNS result should be re-aspirated, but no sooner than 3 months later; the 3-month interval is recommended to prevent false-positive interpretations due to reactive/reparative changes.[11] Ultrasound guidance with immediate, on-site adequacy evaluation is preferred for repeat aspiration after an initial ND/UNS specimen, especially for solid nodules. Repeating the FNA results in a diagnostic interpretation in up to 60% of cases.[12,13] Most nodules with an ND/UNS interpretation prove to be benign.[14,15] After two successive ND/UNS specimens, close clinical follow-up with ultrasound or surgery should be considered, depending upon the clinical findings. Since the risk of malignancy in cystic lesions is low, re-aspiration of most cystic nodules with an initial ND/UNS result should be performed only if the ultrasound findings are suspicious.

Sample Reports

Example 1 (solid nodule):
NONDIAGNOSTIC.
Specimen processed and examined, but nondiagnostic due to insufficient cellularity.
Note: A repeat aspiration should be considered if clinically indicated.

Example 2 (cystic lesion):
NONDIAGNOSTIC.
Cyst fluid only (see Note).
Specimen processed and examined, but nondiagnostic because the specimen consists almost exclusively of histiocytes; interpretation is limited by insufficient follicular cells and/or colloid.
Note: Recommend correlation with cyst size and complexity on ultrasound to assist with further management of the lesion.

Example 3:
UNSATISFACTORY.
Specimen processed and examined, but unsatisfactory due to poor fixation and preservation.
Note: A repeat aspiration should be considered if clinically indicated.

References

1. Oertel YC. Unsatisfactory (vs. nondiagnostic) thyroidal aspirates: a semantic issue? *Diagn Cytopathol*. 2006;34(2):87-88.
2. Baloch ZW, LiVolsi VA, Asa SL, et al. Diagnostic terminology and morphologic criteria for cytologic diagnosis of thyroid lesions: a synopsis of the National Cancer Institute Thyroid Fine-Needle Aspiration State of the Science Conference. *Diagn Cytopathol*. 2008;36(6):425-437.
3. Sudilovsky D. Interpretation of the paucicellular thyroid fine needle aspiration biopsy specimen. *Pathol Case Rev*. 2005;10(2):68-73.
4. Pitman MB, Abele J, Ali SZ, et al. Techniques for thyroid FNA: a synopsis of the National Cancer Institute Thyroid Fine-Needle Aspiration State of the Science Conference. *Diagn Cytopathol*. 2008;36(6):407-424.
5. Jing X, Michael CW, Pu RT. The clinical and diagnostic impact of using standard criteria of adequacy assessment and diagnostic terminology on thyroid nodule fine needle aspiration. *Diagn Cytopathol*. 2008;36(3):161-166.
6. Deshpande V, Kapila K, Sai KS, Verma K. Follicular neoplasms of the thyroid. Decision tree approach using morphologic and morphometric parameters. *Acta Cytol*. 1997;41(2):369-376.
7. Renshaw AA. Evidence-based criteria for adequacy in thyroid fine-needle aspiration. *Am J Clin Pathol*. 2002;118(4):518-521.

8. Choi KU, Kim JY, Park DY, et al. Recommendations for the management of cystic thyroid nodules. *ANZ J Surg.* 2005;75(7):537-541.

9. Nguyen GK, Ginsberg J, Crockford PM. Fine-needle aspiration biopsy cytology of the thyroid. Its value and limitations in the diagnosis and management of solitary thyroid nodules. *Pathol Annu.* 1991;26(Pt 1):63-91.

10. Michael CW, Pang Y, Pu RT, Hasteh F, Griffith KA. Cellular adequacy for thyroid aspirates prepared by ThinPrep: how many cells are needed? *Diagn Cytopathol.* 2007;35(12): 792-797.

11. Layfield LJ, Abrams J, Cochand-Priollet B, et al. Post-thyroid FNA testing and treatment options: a synopsis of the National Cancer Institute Thyroid Fine Needle Aspiration State of the Science Conference. *Diagn Cytopathol.* 2008;36(6):442-448.

12. Orija IB, Pineyro M, Biscotti C, Reddy SS, Hamrahian AH. Value of repeating a nondiagnostic thyroid fine-needle aspiration biopsy. *Endocr Pract.* 2007;13(7):735-742.

13. Alexander EK, Heering JP, Benson CB, et al. Assessment of nondiagnostic ultrasound-guided fine needle aspirations of thyroid nodules. *J Clin Endocrinol Metab.* 2002;87(11): 4924-4927.

14. MacDonald L, Yazdi HM. Nondiagnostic fine needle aspiration biopsy of the thyroid gland: a diagnostic dilemma. *Acta Cytol.* 1996;40(3):423-428.

15. Tamez-Perez HE, Gutierrez-Hermosillo H, Forsbach-Sanchez G, et al. Nondiagnostic thyroid fine needle aspiration cytology: outcome in surgical treatment. *Rev Invest Clin.* 2007;59(3):180-183.

Chapter 3

Benign

Tarik M. Elsheikh, Béatrix Cochand-Priollet,
Pedro Patricio de Agustin, Mary K. Sidawy, and Matthew A. Zarka

Thyroid FNA derives much of its clinical value from its ability to reliably identify benign thyroid nodules, thus sparing many patients with nodular thyroid disease unnecessary surgery. Since most thyroid nodules are benign, a benign result is the most common FNA interpretation (approx. 65% of all cases).[1,2]

To report benign thyroid cytopathology results, the term "Benign" is preferred over other terms such as "Negative for malignancy" and "Non-neoplastic."[3,4] Benign cytopathology is associated with a very low risk of malignancy,[1,5] and patients are usually followed conservatively with periodic clinical and radiologic examinations. Benign results are further sub-classified as benign follicular nodules, thyroiditis, or other less common entities. Nodular goiter (NG) is the most commonly sampled lesion by FNA, and lymphocytic (Hashimoto's) thyroiditis is the most commonly encountered form of thyroiditis.

Benign Follicular Nodule

Background

The benign follicular nodule (BFN) is the most commonly encountered entity in thyroid cytopathology and encompasses a group of benign lesions with similar cytologic features that are classified histologically as nodules in nodular goiter (NG), hyperplastic (adenomatoid) nodules, colloid nodules, nodules in Graves' disease, and a subset of follicular adenomas (those of macrofollicular type). The distinction among these different histologic entities is not possible by FNA, but this is of little importance because they are all benign and, therefore, can be managed in a similar, conservative manner. BFNs are characterized by variable amounts of colloid, benign-appearing follicular cells, Hürthle cells, and macrophages.

Syed Z. Ali and Edmund S. Cibas (eds.), *The Bethesda System for Reporting Thyroid Cytopathology*, DOI 10.1007/978-0-387-87666-5_3,
© Springer Science+Business Media, LLC 2010

Definition

The designation "benign follicular nodule" applies to a cytologic sample that is adequate for evaluation and consists predominantly of colloid and benign-appearing follicular cells in varying proportions. The general term BFN may be utilized in reporting; alternatively, a more specific term like colloid nodule, nodular goiter, hyperplastic/adenomatoid nodule, or Graves' disease may be used, depending on the associated clinical presentation (see Sample Reports).

Criteria (Figs. 3.1–3.13)

Specimens are sparsely to moderately cellular.

Colloid is viscous, shiny, and light yellow or gold in color (resembling honey or varnish) on gross examination. It is dark blue-violet-magenta with Romanowsky-type stains and green to orange-pink with the Papanicolaou stain (Fig. 3.1). It may be thin or thick in texture.

Thin, watery colloid often forms a "thin membrane/cellophane" coating or film with frequent folds that impart a "crazy pavement," "chicken wire," or mosaic appearance (Fig. 3.1).

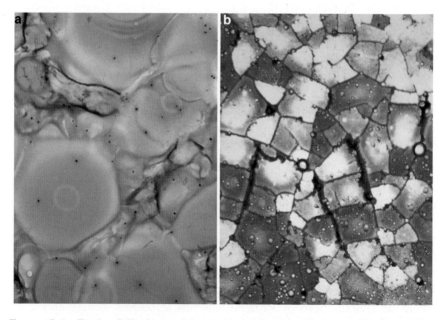

FIGURE 3.1. Benign follicular nodule: watery colloid. a. Watery colloid has a light green-pink color in alcohol-fixed, Papanicolaou-stained preparations and shows a "thin membrane/cellophane coating" appearance (smear, Papanicolaou stain). b. Thick colloid stains dark blue-violet with air-dried, Romanowsky-stained preparations and shows a chicken wire appearance (smear, Diff-Quik stain).

Dense colloid has a hyaline quality and often shows cracks (Fig. 3.2).

Follicular cells are arranged predominantly in monolayered sheets and are evenly spaced ("honeycomb-like") within the sheets (Figs. 3.3, 3.4).

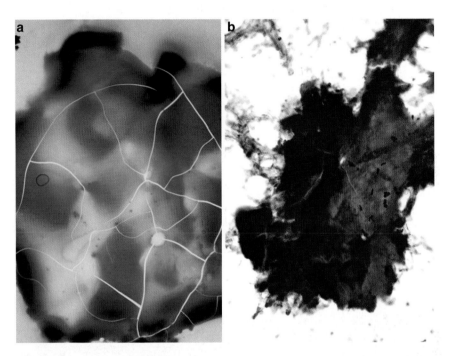

FIGURE 3.2. Benign follicular nodule: thick colloid. a. Thick colloid demonstrates a "stained glass cracking" appearance (smear, Diff-Quik stain). b. Thick colloid appears dense and orange-pink with alcohol-fixed, Papanicolaou-stained preparations (smear, Papanicolaou stain).

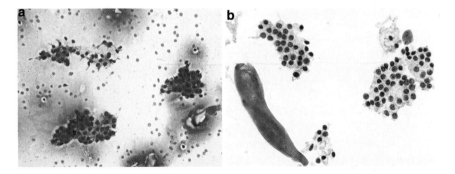

FIGURE 3.3. Benign follicular nodule. Monolayered sheets of evenly spaced follicular cells have a honeycomb-like arrangement. Colloid is observed in the background (a. smear, Diff-Quik stain; b. ThinPrep, Papanicolaou stain).

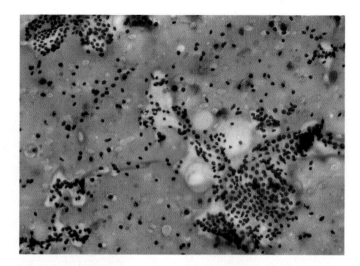

FIGURE 3.4. Benign follicular nodule. Predominantly monolayered sheets of follicular cells are admixed with occasional pigment-laden macrophages. Stripped follicular cell nuclei are present in the background. Orange-pink watery colloid admixed with blood is difficult to recognize in the background (smear, Papanicolaou stain).

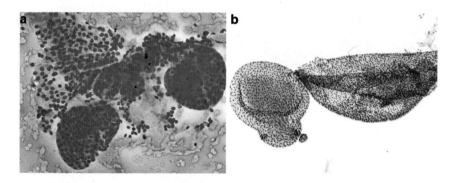

FIGURE 3.5. Benign follicular nodule. Three-dimensional, variably sized balls/spheres are admixed with flat sheets. Within the spheres there is maintenance of polarity, including a relatively evenly spaced nuclear arrangement (a. smear, Diff-Quik stain; b. ThinPrep, Papanicolaou stain).

Occasional follicular cells are arranged in intact, 3-dimensional, variably-sized balls/spheres (Fig. 3.5).

Rare microfollicles may be present.

The follicular cells have scant or moderate amounts of delicate cytoplasm (Figs. 3.6 and 3.7).

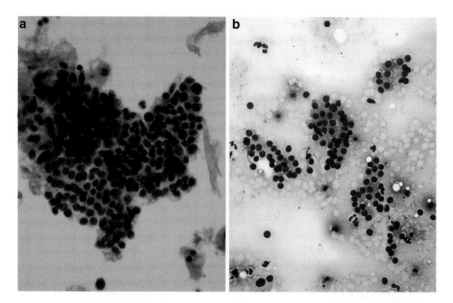

Figure 3.6. Benign follicular nodule. a. Nuclear overlapping in the form of folded sheets may be observed in some clusters (smear, Papanicolaou stain). b. Small flat sheets without significant nuclear overlapping or atypia of follicular cells represent small fragments of macrofollicles, not microfollicles (smear, Diff-Quik stain).

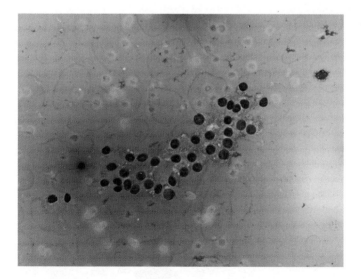

Figure 3.7. Benign follicular nodule. Benign follicular cells have delicate cytoplasm and ill-defined borders. The nuclei are uniformly spaced and approximate the size of red blood cells. Watery colloid is present in the background (smear, Diff-Quik stain).

Follicular cell nuclei are dark, round to oval, approximately the size of a red blood cell, (7–10 microns in diameter), and show a uniformly granular chromatin pattern (Fig. 3.8).

Anisonucleosis is appreciated in some cases, but there is no significant pleomorphism or nuclear atypia.

Minimal nuclear overlapping and crowding can occur (Fig. 3.6).

Green-black cytoplasmic granules may be seen, representing lipofuscin or hemosiderin pigment (Fig. 3.9).

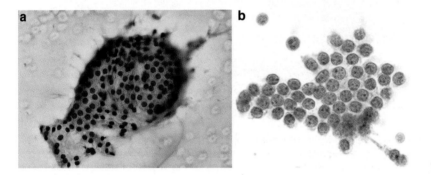

Figure 3.8. Benign follicular nodule. Benign follicular cells have round to oval monomorphic nuclei with finely granular chromatin and inconspicuous to absent nucleoli (a: smear, Papanicolaou stain; b: SurePath preparation, Papanicolaou stain). (The case illustrated in Fig. 3.8B is courtesy of Douglas R. Schneider, MD, Excell Clinical Laboratories, Boston, MA, USA).

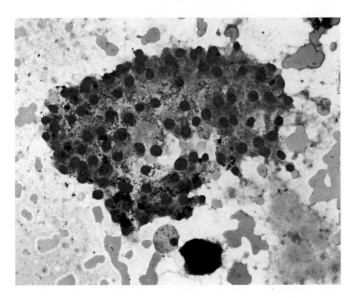

Figure 3.9. Benign follicular nodule. Follicular cells may contain green-black cytoplasmic pigment granules (smear, Diff-Quik stain).

Follicular cells may appear shrunken and degenerated when associated with abundant colloid (Fig. 3.10).

Hürthle cells (oncocytes) are sometimes present, in flat sheets and/or as isolated cells.

Macrophages are commonly present and may contain hemosiderin pigment (Fig. 3.4).

Focal reparative changes are observed, especially in cystic lesions, including cyst lining cells with enlarged nuclei, finely granular chromatin, and a squamoid or spindle-shaped ("tissue-culture cell") appearance (Fig. 3.11).

Explanatory Notes

BFN cytology comprises a morphologically diverse group of benign histologic lesions, ranging from the colloid nodule with minimal cellularity and abundant colloid to the hyperplastic (adenomatoid) nodule with moderate cellularity and scant colloid.[6-9] The predominance of honeycomb-like sheets of follicular cells, admixed in some cases with Hürthle cells, and an abundance of colloid is the hallmark of BFN. Watery colloid is most apparent with one of the Romanowsky-type stains like the commonly used Diff-Quik stain; it is less conspicuous with Papanicolaou-stained preparations (Fig. 3.4).

Watery colloid can be confused with serum in bloody specimens. Helpful clues are the recognition of cracking and folding in colloid, as well as its tendency to surround follicular cells, whereas serum accumulates at the edges of the slide and around platelets, fibrin and blood clots. Specimens

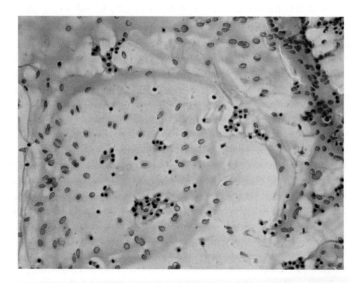

FIGURE 3.10. Benign follicular nodule. Follicular cells may appear shrunken and degenerated when associated with abundant colloid (smear, Papanicolaou stain).

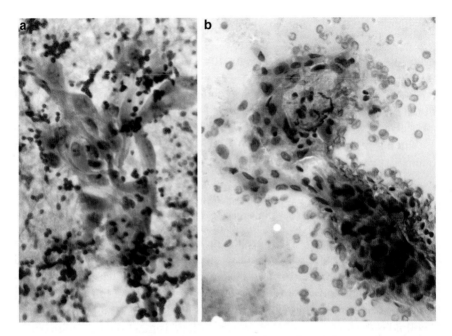

Figure 3.11. Benign follicular nodule: cyst lining cells. a. Reparative changes are commonly associated with cystic degeneration (smear, Papanicolaou stain). b. Occasionally, these cells show nuclear grooves and powdery chromatin. When the changes are focal and mild, particularly if the background is overwhelmingly benign, they are easily recognized as reactive changes, but when more advanced and widespread they raise a concern for papillary carcinoma (smear, Papanicolaou stain).

consisting of abundant colloid only, with very few or no follicular cells, are considered BFNs and may be reported as "suggestive of..." or "consistent with colloid nodule." Under such circumstances, colloid must be distinguished from serum and should cover a significant portion of the glass slide surface (Figs. 3.1, 3.10).

Thyroid cysts with an inadequate number of follicular cells should be interpreted as "Nondiagnostic" or "Unsatisfactory," with a comment pertaining to the "cyst fluid only" nature of the aspirate (see Chap. 2).[10]

Cytoplasmic lipofuscin and hemosiderin pigment granules have no diagnostic significance and can be found in benign and malignant conditions.

Moderately cellular BFNs may prompt consideration of a follicular neoplasm, but cellularity alone is not enough to merit the interpretation "Follicular neoplasm/Suspicious for a follicular neoplasm (FN/SFN)" (Fig. 3.14). Follicular cell crowding, overlapping, and microfollicle formation affecting a majority of the follicular cell population are the important features of the SFN specimen.[11] Some BFNs do contain a minor component of microfollicles. When these comprise a minority of the sample and are outnumbered by macrofollicle fragments, the sample is interpreted as a BFN. Macrofollicle fragments range in size from small to large. A small fragment of benign-appearing follicular cells should not be misconstrued as a microfollicle (Fig. 3.6B): an important defining feature of the microfollicle is the crowding and overlapping of the follicular cells. Similarly, the presence of Hürthle cells per se should not prompt the interpretation "Follicular neoplasm, Hürthle cell type/ Suspicious for a follicular neoplasm, Hürthle cell type (FNHCT/SFNHCT)." A minor population of Hürthle cells is a common finding in BFNs. Less commonly, Hürthle cells can be a prominent or even the predominant component of a BFN, and in some cases there can be significant anisonucleosis and hyperchromasia of the Hürthle cells. The interpretation FNHCT/SFNHCT should be reserved for cases that consist exclusively (or almost exclusively) of Hürthle cells (see Chap. 6).

FNA is unable to distinguish NG from a colloid-rich, macrofollicular adenoma, so the latter will often be diagnosed cytologically as a BFN. Occasionally, an aspirate with the features of a BFN will contain a subpopulation of follicular cells with nuclear features suggestive of papillary thyroid carcinoma (Fig. 3.11). Such cases are interpreted as "Suspicious for malignancy" or "Atypia of Undetermined Significance (AUS)", depending on the extent of atypia (see Chaps. 4 and 7).

The cytologic features and diagnostic accuracy of BFNs are generally similar between smears and liquid-based preparations, but there are a few differences.[12,13] The amount of colloid is diminished in liquid-based preparations when compared with smears, but nuclear detail is superior.[14,15] Benign-appearing follicular cells are arranged in relatively smaller monolayer sheets, usually with less than 20–25 cells per sheet. The cells have pale blue cytoplasm and smaller and darker nuclei (Figs. 3.12, 3.13). Colloid appears as

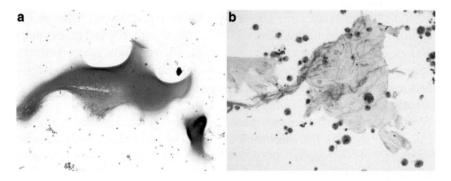

FIGURE 3.12. Benign follicular nodule: colloid (liquid-based preparations). a. Thick colloid on liquid-based preparations resembles its counterpart on smears (SurePath, Papanicolaou stain; case courtesy of Douglas R. Schneider, MD, Excell Clinical Laboratories, Boston, MA, USA). b. Watery colloid has a thin, "tissue-paper" appearance (ThinPrep, Papanicolaou stain).

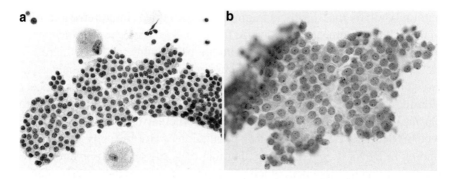

FIGURE 3.13. Benign follicular nodule (liquid-based preparation). The follicular cells have pale cytoplasm and small, round, evenly spaced nuclei. (a. ThinPrep, Papanicolaou stain; b. SurePath, Papanicolaou stain). (The case illustrated in Fig. 3.13B is courtesy of Douglas R. Schneider, MD, Excell Clinical Laboratories, Boston, MA, USA).

either dense, dark blue-orange droplets or thin tissue paper-like sheets.[12] Macrophages may have more abundant pale blue cytoplasm, enlarged, pale nuclei, and prominent nucleoli (Fig. 3.13).

Graves' Disease (Figs. 3.15–3.18)

Graves' disease (GD) is an autoimmune diffuse hyperplastic thyroid disorder, commonly seen in middle-aged women and usually diagnosed clinically due to hyperthyroidism. Most patients have a diffuse rather than nodular enlargement of the thyroid gland and do not require FNA for diagnosis.[16] Occasionally, however, large and/or cold nodules develop that raise the suspicion of a co-existing malignancy and thus prompt FNA. The cytologic features of GD are non-specific, and clinical correlation is needed for a definitive diagnosis. Aspirates are often cellular and show similar features to non-Graves' BFNs, including abundant colloid and a variable number of follicular cells.

Lymphocytes and oncocytes may be seen in the background. Follicular cells are arranged in flat sheets and loosely cohesive groups, with abundant delicate, foamy cytoplasm[17] (Figs. 3.15 and 3.16). Nuclei are often enlarged, vesicular, and show prominent nucleoli. Few microfollicles may be observed. Distinctive flame cells may be prominent, and are represented by marginal cytoplasmic vacuoles with red to pink frayed edges (best appreciated with Romanowsky-type stains)[16] (Fig. 3.15). Flame cells, however, are not specific for GD and may be encountered in other non-neoplastic thyroid conditions, follicular neoplasms, and papillary carcinoma. Occasionally the follicular

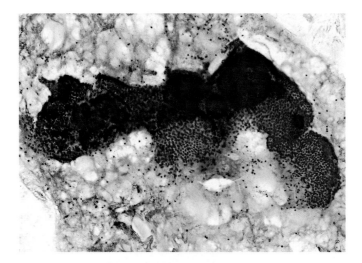

Figure 3.14. Benign follicular nodule. This cellular smear consists predominantly of spheres and large monolayered sheets of follicular cells without significant overlapping or atypia. Colloid was easily recognized elsewhere on the smear (smear, Papanicolaou stain).

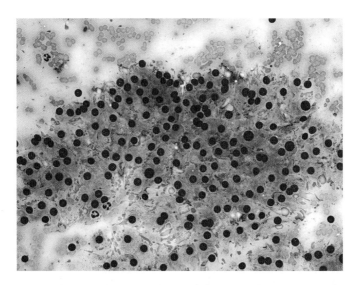

Figure 3.15. Benign follicular nodule (patient with Graves' disease). Large monolayered sheets of cells have abundant cytoplasm. Flame cells are distinctive, and are represented by marginal cytoplasmic vacuoles with red to pink frayed edges (smear, Diff-Quik stain).

cells display focal chromatin clearing and rare intranuclear grooves (Fig. 3.17). These changes are not diffuse, however, and other diagnostic nuclear features of papillary carcinoma are commonly absent.[18] Occasionally, treated GD shows prominent microfollicular architecture, significant nuclear

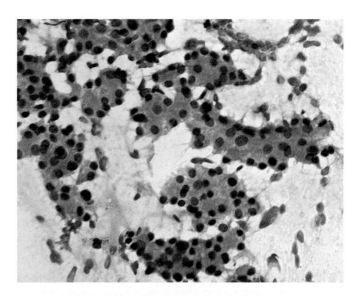

FIGURE 3.16. Benign follicular nodule (patient with Graves' disease). The nuclei are often enlarged, vesicular, and show prominent nucleoli. Anisonucleosis is prominent. The cytoplasm is foamy and delicate in appearance (smear, Papanicolaou stain)

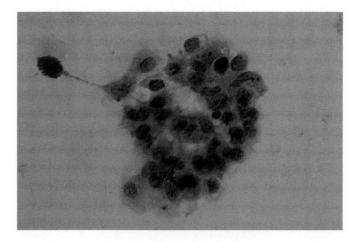

FIGURE 3.17. Benign follicular nodule (patient with Graves' disease). The follicular cells may display focal nuclear chromatin clearing and rare grooves. These changes are rarely diffuse, and other diagnostic nuclear features of papillary carcinoma are absent (smear, Papanicolaou stain).

overlapping and crowding, and considerable atypia. Care must be taken not to over-interpret these changes as malignant or neoplastic, and inquiry should be sought regarding prior radioactive iodine therapy[19] (Fig. 3.18).

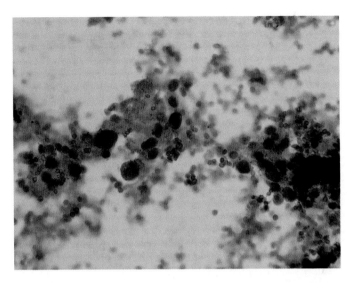

FIGURE 3.18. Benign follicular nodule (patient with Grave's disease after radioactive iodine therapy). There is considerable nuclear crowding and pleomorphism. The atypia, however, has a degenerative quality (smear, Papanicolaou stain).

Lymphocytic (Hashimoto′s) Thyroiditis (Figs. 3.19–3.22)

Background

Lymphocytic thyroiditis (LT) most commonly affects middle-aged women but is also frequent in adolescents. Patients often develop diffuse thyroid enlargement, but become candidates for FNA only when they develop nodularity or an increasing thyroid volume. LT is usually associated with circulating antibodies to thyroglobulin, thyroperoxidase (microsomal antigen), colloid antigen, and thyroid hormones.

Definition

The designation "Consistent with lymphocytic (Hashimoto's) thyroiditis" applies to a cytologic sample composed of many polymorphic lymphoid cells associated with Hürthle cells.[20]

Criteria

Specimens are usually hypercellular, but advanced fibrosis or dilution with blood may decrease the apparent cellularity. An interpretation of lymphocytic

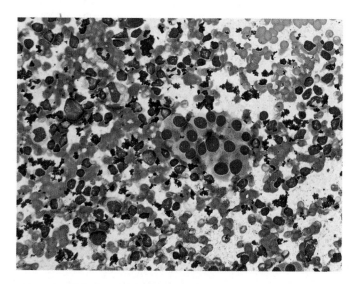

FIGURE 3.19. Lymphocytic (Hashimoto's) thyroiditis. There is a mixed population of Hürthle cells and polymorphic lymphocytes (smear, Diff-Quik stain).

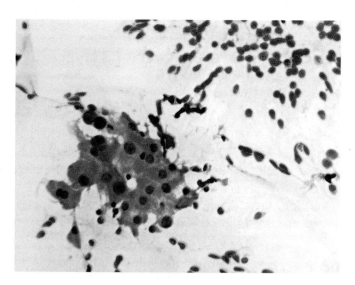

FIGURE 3.20. Lymphocytic (Hashimoto's) thyroiditis. Hürthle cells have abundant granular cytoplatsm, large nuclei, and prominent nucleoli. There is mild anisonucleosis (smear, Papanicolaou stain).

thyroiditis does not require a minimum number of follicular/Hürthle cells for adequacy.[10]

The lymphoid population is polymorphic, including small mature lymphocytes, larger reactive lymphoid cells, and occasional plasma cells.

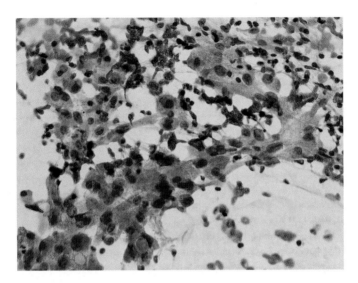

Figure 3.21. Lymphocytic (Hashimoto's) thyroiditis. There is prominent aniso-nucleosis, as well as occasional scattered nuclear grooves. The atypical cells, however, maintain a low nuclear/cytoplasmic ratio and are restricted to areas of inflammation (smear, Papanicolaou stain).

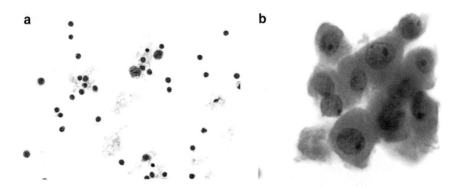

Figure 3.22. Lymphocytic (Hashimoto's) thyroiditis, liquid-based preparations. a. Lymphocytes are dispersed as isolated cells (ThinPrep, Papanicolaou stain). b. Hürthle cells have abundant granular cytoplasm and prominent nucleoli (SurePath, Papanicolaou stain). (The case illustrated in Fig. 3.22B is courtesy of Douglas R. Schneider, MD, Excell Clinical Laboratories, Boston, MA, USA).

The lymphoid cells may be present in the background or infiltrate epithelial cell groups. Intact lymphoid follicles and lymphohistiocytic aggregates may be seen.

Hürthle cells (oncocytes), when present, are arranged in sheets or as isolated cells. They have abundant granular cytoplasm, large nuclei, and prominent nucleoli (Figs 3.19, 3.20).

Anisonucleosis of Hürthle cells may be prominent. Sometimes mild nuclear atypia is encountered, including scattered nuclear clearing and grooves (Figs. 3.21 and 3.22).

Granulomatous (subacute, de Quervain's) Thyroiditis (Fig. 3.23)

Granulomatous (subacute, de Quervain's) thyroiditis is a self-limited inflammatory condition of the thyroid that is usually diagnosed clinically. FNA is generally performed only if there is nodularity that raises the possibility of a co-existing malignancy. In the absence of granulomas, the cytologic findings are nonspecific. The biopsy procedure, however, may be quite painful for the patient, preventing adequate sampling.

Criteria

The cellularity is variable and depends on the stage of disease.

Clusters of epithelioid histiocytes, i.e., granulomas, are present (Fig. 3.23), along with many multinucleated giant cells.

The early stage demonstrates many neutrophils and eosinophils, similar to acute thyroiditis.[21]

In later stages the smears are hypocellular. They show giant cells surrounding and engulfing colloid (Fig. 3.23, inset), epithelioid cells, lymphocytes, macrophages, and scant degenerated follicular cells.[21]

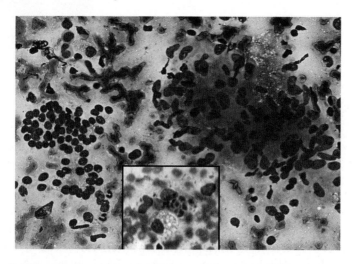

FIGURE 3.23. Granulomatous (subacute) thyroiditis. Epithelioid granulomas, mixed inflammatory cells, and benign follicular cells are present. Inset: Macrophages are seen ingesting colloid (smear, Diff-Quik stain).

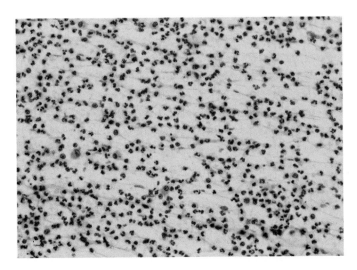

FIGURE 3.24. Acute thyroiditis. There are numerous neutrophils, macrophages, and inflammatory debris (smear, Papanicolaou stain).

In the involutional stage, giant cells and inflammatory cells may be absent; some specimens may be insufficient for evaluation.

Acute Thyroiditis (Fig. 3.24)

Acute thyroiditis is a rare infectious condition of the thyroid, more commonly seen in immunocompromised patients.

Criteria

Numerous neutrophils are associated with necrosis, fibrin, macrophages, and blood.

There are scant reactive follicular cells and limited to absent colloid.

Bacterial or fungal organisms are occasionally seen in the background, especially in immunocompromised patients. Cultures and special stains for organisms may be helpful in these situations.

Riedel's Thyroiditis/Disease (Fig. 3.25)

This is the rarest form of thyroiditis and results in progressive fibrosis of the thyroid gland with extension into the soft tissues of the neck.

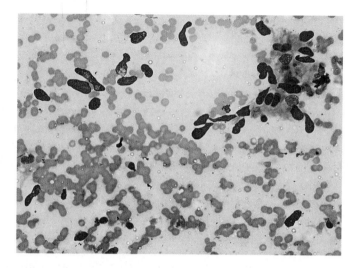

Figure 3.25. Riedel's thyroiditis/disease. The hypocellular smear contains scattered bland spindle cells and rare chronic inflammatory cells (smear, Diff-Quik stain).

Criteria

The thyroid gland feels very firm on palpation.
   The preparations are often acellular.
   Collagen strands and bland spindle cells may be present.
   There are rare chronic inflammatory cells.
   Colloid and follicular cells are usually absent.

Explanatory Notes

In some patients with LT, the predominance of either the lymphoid or the Hürthle cell component may raise the possibility of lymphoma or Hürthle cell neoplasm, respectively.[22,23] A prominent lymphoid population that appears monomorphic should raise the suspicion of lymphoma and prompt additional samples for flow cytometry to confirm the diagnosis (Chap. 12). The diagnosis of FNHCT/SFNHCT should be considered in cases devoid of a lymphocytic infiltrate (Chap. 6). The follicular or Hürthle cells occasionally demonstrate focal reactive changes and mild atypia, including nuclear enlargement, grooves, and chromatin clearing[22] (Fig. 3.21). Therefore, the diagnostic threshold for papillary carcinoma should be raised slightly if there is cytomorphologic evidence of LT. In some cases the features will be equivocal, in which case a diagnosis of AUS or "Suspicious for malignancy" should be considered, depending on how well developed the nuclear changes are. At times, stripped follicular cell nuclei of a BFN may be misinterpreted as lymphocytes (Fig. 3.4); care must be taken to identify the thin rim of cytoplasm surrounding true lymphocytes in order to avoid a false diagnosis of LT (Fig. 3.19).

The diagnosis of LT on liquid-based preparations can be challenging, as the chronic inflammatory background may be decreased or absent.[12,14,24] Since the lymphoid cells tend to be evenly dispersed in the background in liquid-based preparations, they are easy to overlook at low magnification. Liquid-based preparations, which are designed to eliminate red blood cells, are relatively enriched for white blood cells, therefore, care must be taken not to over-interpret the normal lymphocytes of blood as indicative of LT. If the lymphoid cells are present in the normal proportion to neutrophils as seen in peripheral blood, then the lymphoid cells are merely blood elements. In LT, there will be a marked increase in the proportion of lymphoid cells to other inflammatory cells, sometimes accompanied by germinal center fragments. With liquid-based preparations, Hürthle cells occasionally have irregular nuclei.

The cytologic findings are often nonspecific in acute, subacute, and Riedel's thyroiditis, and in some cases there may be an overlap with LT.[20,25] A careful examination of the smears should be undertaken to exclude the possibility of an associated malignancy such as a sclerosing lymphoma or fibrosing anaplastic carcinoma.

Management

Patients with benign thyroid cytology are generally followed clinically with periodic physical examination, supplemented by ultrasonography (US) in some cases.[26,27] Follow-up is carried out at 6–18 month intervals and for at least 3–5 years following the initial benign diagnosis. Repeat FNA is recommended for nodules showing significant growth or developing US abnormalities, such as irregular margins, microcalcifications, intra-nodular hypervascularity, and hypoechogenicity in solid areas.[26]

The risk of cancer associated with cytologically benign thyroid nodules is difficult to calculate because only a minority of nodules with benign cytology (approximately 10%) undergo surgery.[28] A reliable false-negative rate can only be calculated if all patients undergo surgery (gold standard) regardless of their FNA result; this is neither practical nor feasible, however, considering the very low incidence of associated cancer. Most published studies, especially those based on reviews of pooled series, report a false-negative rate in the range of 1–10%.[29–31] However, most of these studies only included surgically resected benign nodules in the calculation and therefore suffered from selection bias. Surgery is recommended only for a selected subset of nodules, including those that are large, symptomatic, have worrisome clinical and/or sonographic characteristics, or are associated with a contralateral malignancy.

A more practical assessment of the false-negative rate can be achieved only from long term (e.g., 5–10 years) clinical follow-up of cytologically benign nodules. There are only a few studies of patients with benign results that were followed long-term, and they have reported a false-negative rate of <1%.[5,32] Ideally, institutions should strive to achieve a false-negative rate that is less than 2–3%.

Sample Reports

If an aspirate is interpreted as Benign, it is implied that the sample is adequate for evaluation. (An explicit statement of adequacy is optional.) Descriptive comments that follow are used to sub-classify the benign interpretation (see examples below). An educational note specifying the risk of malignancy for this interpretation, derived from the experience of the laboratory itself or from the literature, is optional.

Example 1:
  BENIGN.
  Benign follicular nodule.

Example 2:
  BENIGN.
  Benign-appearing follicular cells, colloid, and occasional Hürthle cells, consistent with a benign follicular nodule.

Example 3:
  BENIGN.
  Benign follicular nodule, consistent with colloid nodule.

Example 4:
  BENIGN.
  Consistent with hyperplastic/adenomatoid nodule.

Example 5:
  BENIGN.
  Consistent with colloid nodule.

Example 6 (Clinical history of Hashimoto's thyroiditis provided):
  BENIGN.
  Consistent with lymphocytic (Hashimoto's) thyroiditis.

Example 7 (Not known if the patient has Hashimoto's thyroiditis):
  BENIGN.
  Numerous polymorphic lymphoid cells and scattered Hürthle cells.
  NOTE: The findings are consistent with lymphocytic (Hashimoto's) thyroiditis in the proper clinical setting.

References

1. Yassa L, Cibas ES, Benson CB, et al. Long-term assessment of a multidisciplinary approach to thyroid nodule diagnostic evaluation. *Cancer*. 2007;111(6):508-516.
2. Gharib H, Goellner JR, Johnson DA. Fine-needle aspiration cytology of the thyroid: a 12-year experience with 11, 000 biopsies. *Clin Lab Med*. 1993;13:699-709.
3. Baloch ZW, Cibas ES, Clark DP, et al. The National Cancer Institute Thyroid fine needle aspiration state of the science conference: a summation. *Cytojournal*. 2008;5:6.
4. Baloch ZW, LiVolsi VA, Asa SL, et al. Diagnostic terminology and morphologic criteria for cytologic diagnosis of thyroid lesions: a synopsis of the National Cancer Institute Thyroid Fine-Needle Aspiration State of the Science Conference. *Diagn Cytopathol*. 2008;36(6):425-437.
5. Grant CS, Hay ID, Gough IR, McCarthy PM, Goellner JR. Long-term follow-up of patients with benign thyroid fine-needle aspiration cytologic diagnoses. *Surgery*. 1989;106:980-985.
6. Clark DP, Faquin WC. *Thyroid Cytopathology*. New York: Springer; 2005.
7. Berezowski K, Jovanovic I, Sidawy MK. Thyroid. In: Sidawy MK, Ali SZ, eds. *Fine Needle Aspiration Cytology*. Churchill:Livingstone 2007 [Chapter 2].
8. Elsheikh TM, Singh HK, Saad R, Silverman JF. Fine needle aspiration of the head and neck. In: Barnes L, ed. *Surgical pathology of the head and neck*. New York:Informa Healthcare USA 2009.
9. Orell SR, Philips J. *The Thyroid. Fine needle biopsy and cytological diagnosis of thyroid lesions*. Vols. 14. Basel:Kaarger 1997.
10. Pitman MB, Abele J, Ali S, et al. Techniques for Thyroid FNA: a synopsis of the national cancer institute thyroid fine needle aspiration state of the science conference. *Diagn Cytopathol*. 2008;36(6):407-424.
11. Suen KC. How does one separate cellular follicular lesions of the thyroid by fine-needle aspiration biopsy? *Diagn Cytopathol*. 1988;4:78-81.
12. Tulecke MA, Wang HH. ThinPrep for cytologic evaluation of follicular thyroid lesions: correlation with histologic findings. *Diagn Cytopathol*. 2004;30(1):7-13.
13. Hoda RS. Non-gynecologic cytology on liquid-based preparations: A morphologic review of facts and artifacts. *Diagn Cytopathol*. 2007;35(10):621-634.
14. Cochand-Priollet B, Prat JJ, Polivka M, Thienpont L, Dahan H, Wassef M, et al. Thyroid fine needle aspiration: the morphological features on ThinPrep slide preparations. Eighty cases with histological control. *Cytopathology* 2003;14(6):343–349.
15. Malle D, Valeri RM, Pazaitou-Panajiotou K, Kiziridou A, Vainas I, Destouni C. Use of a thin-layer technique in thyroid fine needle aspiration. *Acta Cytol*. 2006;50(1):23-27.
16. Soderstrom N, Nilsson G. Cytologic diagnosis of thyrotoxicosis. *Acta Med Scand*. 1979;205(4):263-265.
17. Baloch ZW, Sack MJ, Yu GH, Livolsi VA, Gupta PK. Fine-needle aspiration of thyroid: an institutional experience. *Thyroid*. 1998;8(7):565-569.
18. Anderson SR, Mandel S, LiVolsi VA, Gupta PK, Baloch ZW. Can cytomorphology differentiate between benign nodules and tumors arising in Graves' disease? *Diagn Cytopathol*. 2004;31(1):64-67.
19. Centeno BA, Szyfelbein WM, Daniels GH, Vickery AL. Fine-needle aspiration biopsy of the thyroid gland in patients with prior Graves' disease treated with radioactive iodine: morphologic findings and potential pitfalls. *Acta Cytol*. 1996;40:1189-1197.
20. Jayaram G, Marwaha RK, Gupta RK, Sharma SK. Cytomorphologic aspects of thyroiditis. A study of 51 cases with functional, immunologic and ultrasonographic data. *Acta Cytol* 1987;31(6):687–693.

21. Lu CP, Chang TC, Wang CY, Hsiao YL. Serial changes in ultrasound-guided fine needle aspiration cytology in subacute thyroiditis. *Acta Cytol.* 1997;41(2):238-243.
22. Kumarasinghe MP, De Silva S. Pitfalls in cytological diagnosis of autoimmune thyroiditis. *Pathology.* 1999;31(1):1-7.
23. MacDonald L, Yazdi HM. Fine needle aspiration biopsy of Hashimoto's thyroiditis. Sources of diagnostic error. Acta Cytol 1999;43(3):400-6.
24. Frost AR, Sidawy MK, Ferfelli M, et al. Utility of thin-layer preparations in thyroid fine-needle aspiration. Diagnostic accuracy, cytomorphology, and optimal sample preparation. *Cancer* (Cancer Cytopathol) 1998;84:17–25.
25. Harigopal M, Sahoo S, Recant WM, DeMay RM. Fine-needle aspiration of Riedel's disease: report of a case and review of the literature. *Diagn Cytopathol.* 2004;30(3):193-197.
26. Layfield L, Cochand-Priollet B, LiVolsi V, Abrams J, Merino M, Gharib H. *et al.* Post Thyroid FNA Testing and Treatment Options: A synopsis of the national cancer institute thyroid fine needle aspiration state of the science conference. Diagnostic Cytopathology; 2008.
27. Cooper DS, Doherty GM, Haugen BR, et al. Management guidelines for patients with thyroid nodules and differentiated thyroid cancer. *Thyroid.* 2006;16(2):109-142.
28. Bakhos R, Selvaggi SM, DeJong S, et al. Fine-needle aspiration of the thyroid: rate and causes of cytohistopathologic discordance. *Diagn Cytopathol.* 2000;23(4):233-237.
29. Gharib H, Goellner JR. Fine-needle aspiration biopsy of the thyroid: an appraisal. *Ann Int Med.* 1993;118:282-289.
30. Yeh MW, Demircan O, Ituarte P, Clark OH. False-negative fine-needle aspiration cytology results delay treatment and adversely affect outcome in patients with thyroid carcinoma. *Thyroid.* 2004;14(3):207-215.
31. Tee YY, Lowe AJ, Brand CA, Judson RT. Fine-needle aspiration may miss a third of all malignancy in palpable thyroid nodules: a comprehensive literature review. *Ann Surg.* 2007;246(5):714-720.
32. Liel Y, Ariad S, Barchana M. Long-term follow-up of patients with initially benign thyroid fine-needle aspirations. *Thyroid.* 2001;11(8):775-778.

Chapter 4

Atypia of Undetermined Significance/Follicular Lesion of Undetermined Significance

Jeffrey F. Krane, Ritu Nayar, and Andrew A. Renshaw

Background

The classification of "indeterminate" lesions (those not clearly benign or malignant) in thyroid cytopathology has long been a source of confusion for both pathologists and clinicians. There has been much variation in how cytopathologists perceive, interpret, and report such aspirates, especially when the uncertainty relates to follicular lesions. Clinicians have tended to lump interpretations like "follicular lesion," "atypical," "follicular neoplasm," "indeterminate for neoplasia," and "suspicious for malignancy" into a single "indeterminate for malignancy" category for conceptual and even management purposes.[1,2] Follow up studies, however, have shown significantly different clinical outcomes for distinct subcategories within the generic indeterminate category.[3-5] For this reason, it is advisable to define and distinguish categories with distinct risk associations for malignancy, like "Suspicious for follicular neoplasm" versus "Suspicious for malignancy (e.g., papillary carcinoma)."[6,7] In a minority of cases, the cytologic and/or architectural atypia encountered is of uncertain significance: it is of an insufficient degree to qualify for any of the suspicious categories. Such cases have a lower risk of malignancy and deserve to be separated from the suspicious categories.[4,7-9]

Definition

The general diagnostic category "Atypia of Undetermined Significance" (AUS) is reserved for specimens that contain cells (follicular, lymphoid, or other) with architectural and/or nuclear atypia that is not sufficient to be classified as suspicious for a follicular neoplasm, suspicious for malignancy, or malignant. On the other hand, the atypia is more marked than can be

Syed Z. Ali and Edmund S. Cibas (eds.), *The Bethesda System for Reporting Thyroid Cytopathology*, DOI 10.1007/978-0-387-87666-5_4,
© Springer Science+Business Media, LLC 2010

ascribed confidently to benign changes. A contributing factor to the uncertainty is often (but not always) a compromised specimen, e.g., one that is sparsely cellular or obscured by blood or excessive clotting. The term "Follicular Lesion of Undetermined Significance (FLUS)" is equally acceptable for the great majority of cases in which the atypia is of follicular origin (i.e., not lymphoid or other). In general, the clinical approach to a nodule with an initial AUS/FLUS interpretation is a repeat biopsy after a reasonable interval, although in specific clinical settings other management options may be more appropriate.

Criteria (Figs 4.1–4.8)

The heterogeneity of this category precludes outlining all scenarios for which an AUS interpretation is appropriate. The most common situations, however, are outlined here.

1. There is a prominent population of microfollicles in an aspirate that does not otherwise fulfill the criteria for "Follicular Neoplasm/Suspicious for Follicular Neoplasm." This situation may arise when a predominance of microfollicles are seen in a sparsely cellular aspirate with scant colloid. Alternatively, a more prominent than usual population of microfollicles may occur (and may be disproportionately apparent on a minority of smears) in a moderately or markedly cellular sample, but the overall proportion of microfollicles is not sufficient for a diagnosis of "Follicular Neoplasm/Suspicious for Follicular Neoplasm."
2. There is a predominance of Hürthle cells in a sparsely cellular aspirate with scant colloid.
3. Interpretation of follicular cell atypia is hindered by sample preparation artifact, e.g.,
   a. Air-drying artifact with slight nuclear and cytoplasmic enlargement, pale and slightly smudgy chromatin, and/or mildly irregular nuclear contours.
   b. Clotting artifact with apparent cellular crowding.
4. A moderately or markedly cellular sample is composed of a virtually exclusive population of Hürthle cells, yet the clinical setting suggests a benign Hürthle cell nodule:
   a. Lymphocytic (Hashimoto) thyroiditis
   b. Multinodular goiter (MNG)
5. There are focal features suggestive of papillary carcinoma, including nuclear grooves, enlarged nuclei with pale chromatin, and alterations in nuclear contour and shape in an otherwise predominantly benign-appearing sample (especially in patients with Hashimoto thyroiditis or those with abundant colloid and other benign-appearing follicular cells).

6. There are cyst-lining cells which may appear atypical due to the presence of nuclear grooves, prominent nucleoli, elongated nuclei and cytoplasm, and/or intranuclear cytoplasmic inclusions in an otherwise predominantly benign-appearing sample.
7. A minor population of follicular cells show nuclear enlargement, often accompanied by prominent nucleoli.
   a. Specimens from patients with a history of radioactive iodine, carbimazole, or other pharmaceutical agents
   b. Repair due to involutional changes such as cystic degeneration and or hemorrhage
8. There is an atypical lymphoid infiltrate (in which a repeat aspirate for flow cytometry is desirable), but the degree of atypia is insufficient for the general category "suspicious for malignancy."
9. Not otherwise categorized.

Explanatory Notes

An AUS result has been reported in 3–18% of thyroid FNAs.[4,5,8,10] Despite the efforts herein to define this category and provide specific criteria, the use of this category by different pathologists will vary, and AUS can be expected to have, at best, only fair reproducibility. With these caveats in mind, as a provisional goal for most practice settings, the frequency of AUS interpretations should be in the range of approximately 7% of all thyroid FNA interpretations. This figure may be further refined as more laboratories report their experiences using the AUS designation within the context of these criteria.

AUS is a category of last resort and should not be used indiscriminately. For example, the mere presence of some Hürthle cells or cyst-lining cells, with their customary mild nuclear alterations (e.g., nuclear grooves, finely granular or pale chromatin), does not warrant an AUS designation if there is ample evidence of benign follicular cells and abundant colloid. Isolated follicular cells with minimal alterations (isolated nuclear enlargement, pale chromatin, or nuclear grooves) or occasional microfollicles also do not merit the AUS category.

AUS specimens may be compromised in some fashion that precludes a more definitive classification, often because of sparse cellularity. A common example is the sparsely cellular aspirate with a predominance of crowded follicular cells in microfollicular or trabecular arrangements ("architectural atypia") (Fig. 4.1). In a moderately-to-markedly cellular specimen, most samples with a predominance of follicular cells in crowded microfollicular or trabecular groups merit the interpretation "Follicular Neoplasm/

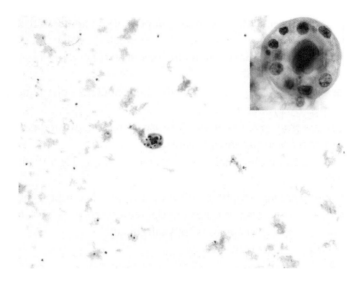

Figure 4.1. Atypia of Undetermined Significance. Scanning magnification reveals a sparsely cellular specimen with a predominance of microfollicles. (Inset: high magnification of a microfollicle) (ThinPrep, Papanicolaou stain).

Suspicious for a Follicular Neoplasm" (see Chap. 5). In general, cytologists are reluctant to make that interpretation on a sparsely cellular sample because the lesion may not have been properly sampled. A similar example is the sparsely cellular aspirate that is comprised exclusively of Hürthle cells. In a moderately or markedly cellular specimen, a sample that consists entirely of Hürthle cells usually merits the interpretation "Follicular Neoplasm, Hürthle cell type/Suspicious for a Follicular Neoplasm, Hürthle cell type (FNHCT/SFNHCT)" (see Chap. 6). Most cytologists, again, are reluctant to make that interpretation on a sparsely cellular sample because of sampling concerns.

Specimen preparation artifacts also account for some instances of AUS. Inadvertent air drying of alcohol-fixed, Papanicolaou (or hematoxylin and eosin) stained smears may result in follicular cells with enlarged nuclei that have pale but slightly smudgy chromatin and irregular nuclear outlines (Fig. 4.2). These features can raise the possibility of papillary carcinoma. Excessive blood clotting can impair the presentation of follicular cells, often giving the false impression of architectural crowding due to the entrapment of cells in the clot or nuclear grooves due to fibrin strands (Fig. 4.3). If the artifacts described above are focal, clearly recognizable, and associated with benign material elsewhere, such cases should be diagnosed as benign. Alternatively, when the artifacts are so pervasive as to preclude fulfilling standard adequacy criteria for well preserved follicular cells, such aspirates should be deemed unsatisfactory for evaluation. In some cases, however, it

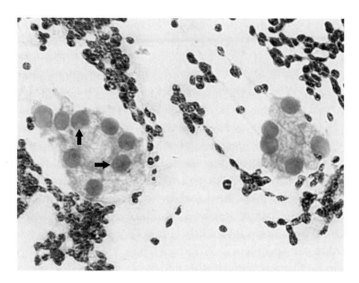

FIGURE 4.2. Atypia of Undetermined Significance. Inadvertent air drying of alcohol-fixed smears leads to suboptimal nuclear detail (e.g., artifactual pallor, enlargement). Such changes mimic subtle features of papillary carcinoma, leading to uncertainty in diagnosis. Note the poorly-defined, possible nuclear pseudoinclusions (arrows) (smear, Papanicolaou stain).

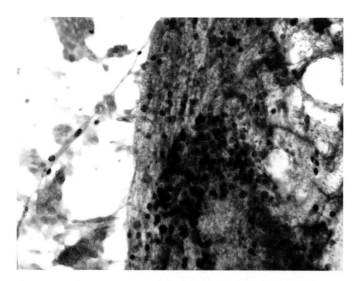

FIGURE 4.3. Atypia of Undetermined Significance. Extensive blood and clotting can distort the arrangement of follicular cells and make them look artifactually crowded. When crowded groups predominate, they raise the possibility of a follicular neoplasm, but extensive clotting raises uncertainty about the findings. The distinction between a "Nondiagnostic" and an AUS specimen rests on the judgment of the cytopathologist based on an assessment of the entire sample and the extent of the artifact (smear, Papanicolaou stain).

is difficult to be sure that the cytologic changes are entirely artifactual in origin, and in such cases AUS is an appropriate diagnosis. The possibility of artifactual changes should be acknowledged in reporting these specimens.

A moderately or markedly cellular aspirate from a solitary nodule that is composed virtually exclusively of Hürthle cells is reported as FNHCT/SFNHCT. In some clinical settings, namely Hashimoto thyroiditis and MNG, this pattern is believed to be more highly predictive of a hyperplastic Hürthle cell nodule (and less predictive of a Hürthle cell neoplasm) than usual. It is thus acceptable to diagnose an exclusively Hürthle cell specimen in a patient with MNG as AUS (see Chap. 6). If interpreted as AUS, an explanatory note that raises the possibility of a Hürthle cell hyperplasia can be very helpful (see Sample Report 6). Similarly, in a patient known to have lymphocytic (Hashimoto) thyroiditis, it is acceptable to diagnose an exclusively Hürthle cell specimen as AUS (see Chap. 6). If interpreted as AUS, a note explaining that a benign Hürthle cell hyperplasia is favored can be very helpful (see Sample Report 7). The note that accompanies an AUS interpretation in this setting is meant to more accurately reflect the underlying risk of malignancy, which, although not well characterized, is considered to be lower than that of FNHCT/SFNHCT in general. The goal is to provide the clinician with the opportunity to avoid an unnecessary lobectomy in some of these patients. In this setting, the clinical decision to follow a patient rather than perform a lobectomy will often be based on clinical and sonographic correlation; it is not clear whether a repeat aspiration – the usual management for an AUS nodule - is likely to add any helpful information.

Separation of the AUS category from suspicious for malignancy is more problematic in aspirates with focal features of papillary carcinoma. A pattern diagnosed by some cytologists as atypical with a qualifier that papillary carcinoma cannot be ruled out is associated with papillary carcinoma in approximately 30–40% of cases.[11,12] As described, this pattern has rare cells (typically less than 20 in number[11]) with enlarged, often overlapping nuclei with pale chromatin, irregular nuclear outlines, and nuclear grooves. When accompanied by even rare, well-defined, intranuclear inclusions and/or psammomatous calcifications, these findings are even more highly associated with papillary carcinoma.[12] A second pattern highly associated with the follicular variant of papillary carcinoma is characterized by diffuse but subtle nuclear enlargement, nuclear irregularity, and only occasional intranuclear grooves, sometimes associated with a microfollicular architecture.[13] Because both of these patterns are highly associated with papillary carcinoma, such aspirates are better classified as suspicious for malignancy (see Chap. 7) or suspicious for a follicular neoplasm (see Chap. 5). The AUS designation should be reserved for those rare cases with few cells with distinct but mildly atypical nuclear features (Fig. 4.4 and 4.5), something which

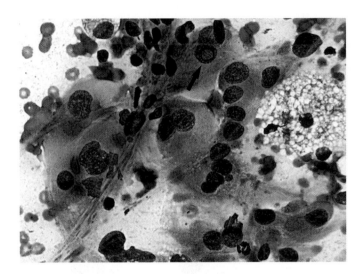

FIGURE 4.4. Atypia of Undetermined Significance (patient with history of Hashimoto's thyroiditis). Oncocytic follicular cells show nuclear enlargement and rare nuclear pseudoinclusions (arrow) (smear, Diff-Quik stain).

can occur in some cases of Hashimoto thyroiditis (see Chap. 3, "Benign") but also in macrofollicular papillary carcinomas. It must be acknowledged that this distinction may be difficult; pathologist experience influences the recognition and correct classification of these cases. Expert consultation may be warranted especially in challenging cases.

Cyst-lining cells are reactive follicular/mesenchymal cells associated with cystic degeneration of thyroid nodules. As such, they have very characteristic features and can be diagnosed as benign in most cases.[14] These cells are typically elongated, with pale chromatin, occasional intranuclear grooves, and relatively large nucleoli, and are virtually always associated with hemosiderin-laden macrophages. The spindle-shaped morphology of the cell and nucleus, reminiscent of reparative epithelium in cervical, bronchial, and gastrointestinal cytologic specimens, is helpful in distinguishing these cells from papillary carcinoma. In some cases, however, the cells are more closely packed, less elongated, and, as a result, more difficult to distinguish definitively from papillary carcinoma (Fig. 4.6).[14] In such cases a diagnosis of AUS is appropriate.

Isolated nuclear enlargement, typically with prominent nucleoli, is common in benign thyroid nodules and by itself does not indicate malignancy. In patients treated with radioactive iodine, carbimazole, or other pharmaceutical agents, nuclear enlargement can be especially prominent.[15–17] When the changes are mild and characteristic in a specimen accompanied by a clinical history of such treatment, a benign interpretation can often be rendered.

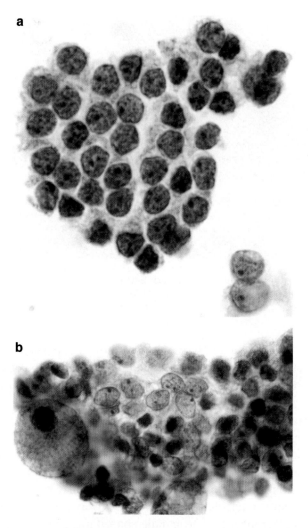

FIGURE 4.5. Atypia of Undetermined Significance. (**a**) Most of the follicular cells are arranged in benign-appearing macrofollicle fragments. (**b**) Rare cells have pale nuclei and mildly irregular nuclear membranes. When such cells are few in number, an atypical interpretation is more appropriate than "suspicious for malignancy" (ThinPrep, Papanicolaou stain).

In some patients, however, the changes can be extreme and raise the possibility of papillary carcinoma or other malignancy (Fig. 4.7).[16,17] In such cases, an AUS interpretation is warranted.

Most AUS cases are based on follicular cell atypia, but in rare cases the AUS designation may be appropriate for a non-follicular and even non-epithelial atypia. An example of non-epithelial atypia that may warrant

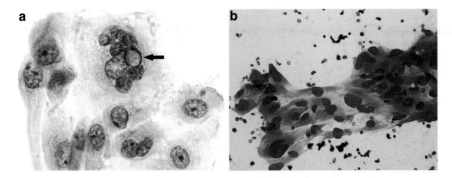

FIGURE 4.6. Atypia of Undetermined Significance. (**a**) In this sparsely cellular specimen, some of the cells had abundant cytoplasm and enlarged nuclei, some with prominent nucleoli. One nucleus has an apparent intranuclear pseudoinclusion (arrow). Such changes may represent atypical but benign cyst lining cells, but a papillary carcinoma cannot be entirely excluded (ThinPrep, Papanicolaou stain). (**b**) Reparative changes in cyst lining cells can mimic some cytologic features of papillary carcinoma (smear, Romanowsky stain).

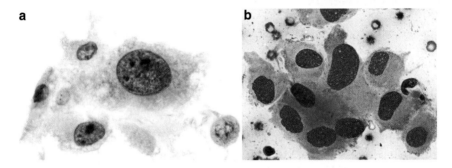

FIGURE 4.7. Atypia of Undetermined Significance. (**a**) These follicular cells, in a patient with Graves' disease treated with methimazole (Tapazole®), show marked nuclear enlargement and anisonucleosis. (ThinPrep, Papanicolaou stain.) (**b**) These atypical follicular cells were obtained from a patient with a history of ionizing radiation to the neck (smear, Romanowsky stain).

the AUS category is an atypical or monomorphous lymphoid infiltrate, especially in the setting of longstanding Hashimoto thyroiditis. In some cases, the findings are not sufficiently concerning to warrant a suspicious or positive for malignancy diagnosis. Aspirates that have a prominent, somewhat polymorphous lymphoid component may raise concern for an extranodal marginal zone B-cell lymphoma (Fig. 4.8). If clonality studies are not available, an AUS diagnosis, with a recommendation for a repeat aspirate for flow cytometry, is appropriate.

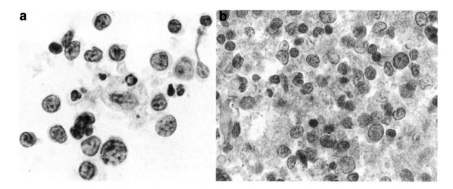

Figure 4.8. Atypia of Undetermined Significance. (**a**) The sample is composed of a heterogeneous infiltrate of lymphoid cells, including occasional atypical forms. There is a tingible body macrophage in the center of the field. Clonality studies were not available in this case. (ThinPrep, Papanicolaou stain.) (**b**) The cell block shows similar features (hematoxylin and eosin stain).

Management

The recommended management for an initial AUS interpretation is the clinical correlation and, for most cases, a repeat FNA at an appropriate interval.[4,18] A repeat FNA usually results in a more definitive interpretation; only about 20–25% of nodules are repeatedly AUS.[4,5] The risk of malignancy for an AUS nodule is difficult to ascertain because only a subset of cases in this category have surgical follow-up. Those that are resected represent a selected population of patients with repeatedly AUS results or patients with worrisome clinical or sonographic findings. In this selected population, 20–25% of patients with AUS prove to have cancer after surgery, but this is undoubtedly an overestimate for all AUS nodules.[4,8] Extrapolating for all AUS nodules (including those patients with negative follow-up in whom surgery was not performed), the risk of malignancy is probably closer to 5–15%.

Sample Reports

If an aspirate is interpreted as AUS, it is implied that the sample is adequate for evaluation. (An explicit statement of adequacy is optional.) Narrative comments that follow are used to further describe the findings. In the narrative comments, some cytologists may prefer to avoid phrases associated with malignancy (e.g., "pseudoinclusions," "pale chromatin," "microfollicles") and substitute generic descriptors (e.g., "focal cytologic atypia," "architectural atypia") to avoid confusion with the suspicious categories, which may prompt surgery rather than the intended more conservative management.

A differential diagnosis and a recommendation can be especially helpful for cases that fall into the AUS category.

Example 1:
ATYPIA OF UNDETERMINED SIGNIFICANCE.
Sparsely cellular aspirate comprised of follicular cells with architectural atypia. Colloid is absent.
Note: A repeat aspirate after an appropriate interval of observation may be helpful if clinically indicated.

Example 2:
ATYPIA OF UNDETERMINED SIGNIFICANCE.
Follicular cells with focal cytologic and architectural atypia, but obscuring blood and clotting artifact preclude definitive evaluation.
Note: A repeat aspirate after an appropriate interval of observation might be helpful if clinically indicated.

Example 3:
ATYPIA OF UNDETERMINED SIGNIFICANCE.
Follicular cells, predominantly benign-appearing, with focal cytologic atypia.
Note: A repeat aspirate after an appropriate interval of observation might be helpful if clinically indicated.

Example 4:
ATYPIA OF UNDETERMINED SIGNIFICANCE.
Predominantly benign-appearing follicular cells; some show focal cytologic and architectural atypia.
Note: A repeat aspirate after an appropriate interval of observation may be helpful if clinically indicated.

Example 5:
FOLLICULAR LESION OF UNDETERMINED SIGNIFICANCE.

Example 6 (FNA of a nodule in the right lobe in a patient with multiple nodules):
ATYPIA OF UNDETERMINED SIGNIFICANCE.
The specimen is moderately cellular and consists almost exclusively of Hürthle cells. Colloid is scant, and there is no apparent increase in lymphoid cells.
Note: In a patient with multiple nodules, the findings likely represent a Hürthle cell hyperplasia in the setting of multinodular goiter, but a Hürthle cell neoplasm cannot be entirely excluded. Clinical correlation is advised.

Example 7 (FNA of a nodule in a patient with a history of Hashimoto thyroiditis):

ATYPIA OF UNDETERMINED SIGNIFICANCE.
The sample consists exclusively of Hürthle cells.
Note: In a patient with Hashimoto thyroiditis, the findings likely represent a Hürthle cell hyperplasia, but a Hürthle cell neoplasm cannot be entirely excluded. Clinical correlation is advised.

Example 8 (FNA of a nodule in a patient treated with ^{131}I):
ATYPIA OF UNDETERMINED SIGNIFICANCE.
Marked cytologic atypia of follicular cells.
Note: In a patient treated with radioiodine, the findings likely represent reactive, treatment-related changes, but a neoplasm cannot be entirely excluded. Clinical correlation is advised.

Example 9:
ATYPIA OF UNDETERMINED SIGNIFICANCE.
Numerous relatively monomorphic lymphoid cells.
Note: The findings are atypical and raise the possibility of a lymphoproliferative lesion, but immunophenotyping studies could not be performed because of insufficient material. An additional aspiration, with apportioning of fresh needle-rinse fluid for flow cytometry, might be helpful if clinically indicated.

References

1. Cooper DS, Doherty GM, Haugen BR, et al. Management guidelines for patients with thyroid nodules and differentiated thyroid cancer. *Thyroid.* 2006;16(2):109-142.
2. Wang HH. Reporting thyroid fine-needle aspiration: literature review and a proposal. *Diagn Cytopathol.* 2006;34(1):67-76.
3. Gharib H, Goellner JR, Johnson DA. Fine-needle aspiration cytology of the thyroid: a 12-year experience with 11, 000 biopsies. *Clin Lab Med.* 1993;13:699-709.
4. Yassa L, Cibas ES, Benson CB, et al. Long-term assessment of a multidisciplinary approach to thyroid nodule diagnostic evaluation. *Cancer.* 2007;111(6):508-516.
5. Nayar R, Ivanovic M. The indeterminate thyroid FNA: Experience from an academic center using terminology similar to that proposed in the 2007 NCI Thyroid Fine Needle Aspiration State of the Science Conference. *Cancer Cytopathol* 2009;117:195–202.
6. Gharib H, Goellner JR. Fine-needle aspiration biopsy of the thyroid: an appraisal. *Ann Int Med.* 1993;118:282-289.
7. Baloch ZW, LiVolsi VA, Asa SL, et al. Diagnostic terminology and morphologic criteria for cytologic diagnosis of thyroid lesions: a synopsis of the National Cancer Institute Thyroid Fine-Needle Aspiration State of the Science Conference. *Diagn Cytopathol.* 2008;36(6):425-437.
8. Yang J, Schnadig V, Logrono R, Wasserman PG. Fine-needle aspiration of thyroid nodules: a study of 4703 patients with histologic and clinical correlations. *Cancer.* 2007;111(5):306-315.
9. Poller DN, Ibrahim AK, Cummings MH, et al. Fine-needle aspiration of the thyroid; the importance of an indeterminate diagnostic category. *Cancer (Cancer Cytopathol).* 2000;90:239-244.

10. Renshaw AA. Accuracy of thyroid fine-needle aspiration using receiver operator characteristic curves. *Am J Clin Pathol.* 2001;116:477-482.
11. Renshaw AA. Focal features of papillary carcinoma of the thyroid in fine-needle aspiration material are strongly associated with papillary carcinoma at resection. *Am J Clin Pathol.* 2002;118(2):208-210.
12. Weber D, Brainard J, Chen L. Atypical epithelial cells, cannot exclude papillary carcinoma, in fine needle aspiration of the thyroid. *Acta Cytol.* 2008;52(3):320-324.
13. Logani S, Gupta PK, LiVolsi VA, et al. Thyroid nodules with FNA cytology suspicious for follicular variant of papillary thyroid carcinoma: follow-up and management. *Diagn Cytopathol.* 2000;23(6):380-385.
14. Faquin WC, Cibas ES, Renshaw AA. "Atypical" cells in fine-needle aspiration biopsy specimens of benign thyroid cysts. *Cancer.* 2005;105(2):71-79.
15. Smejkal V, Smejkalova E, Rosa M, et al. Cytologic changes simulating malignancy in thyrotoxic goiters treated with carbimazole. *Acta Cytol.* 1985;29:173-178.
16. Granter SR, Cibas ES. Cytologic findings in thyroid nodules after 131iodine treatment of hyperthyroidism. *Am J Clin Pathol.* 1997;107:20-25.
17. Centeno BA, Szyfelbein WM, Daniels GH, et al. Fine-needle aspiration biopsy of the thyroid gland in patients with prior Graves' disease treated with radioactive iodine: morphologic findings and potential pitfalls. *Acta Cytol.* 1996;40:1189-1197.
18. Layfield LJ, Abrams J, Cochand-Priollet B, et al. Post-thyroid FNA testing and treatment options: a synopsis of the National Cancer Institute Thyroid Fine Needle Aspiration State of the Science Conference. *Diagn Cytopathol.* 2008;36(6):442-448.

Chapter 5

Follicular Neoplasm/Suspicious for a Follicular Neoplasm

Michael R. Henry, Richard M. DeMay, and Katherine Berezowski

Background

There has been great variability in the way thyroid aspirates that are suspicious for a follicular neoplasm have been reported, as demonstrated by a review of the literature compiled for the NCI-sponsored State of the Science Conference in 2007.[1] The terminology used has ranged from broad terms like "follicular lesion," "follicular proliferation," and "indeterminate" to the more specific terms like "rule out/suggestive of/suspicious for follicular neoplasm" to the definitive "follicular neoplasm."[2–10] Much of this variability results from the fact that the so-called "follicular lesions," comprised of nodular goiter (nodular hyperplasia), follicular adenoma, and follicular carcinoma, have overlapping cytomorphologic features and cannot be accurately distinguished by fine needle aspiration (FNA) alone. Nevertheless, certain cytologic features are very useful in raising the possibility of a neoplasm, most importantly the possibility of a follicular carcinoma. In this regard, FNA can be considered a screening test, selecting for surgery those nodules with a greater probability of malignancy. The final diagnosis depends upon lobectomy because capsular and/or vascular invasion are the *sine qua non* of follicular carcinoma.

In the Bethesda System, the terms "Follicular Neoplasm" and "Suspicious for Follicular neoplasm" are equally acceptable for this category. "Suspicious for a follicular neoplasm (SFN)" is preferred over "Follicular neoplasm (FN)" by some laboratories because a significant proportion (up to 35%) of cases that fulfill the criteria described herein prove not to be neoplasms but rather hyperplastic proliferations in nodular goiter.[3–5,11,12] The term SFN acknowledges this limitation, provides a rational framework for cytologic-histologic correlation, and preserves the credibility of cytopathologists with their clinical colleagues and the patients they serve. This limitation of current thyroid FNA

Syed Z. Ali and Edmund S. Cibas (eds.), *The Bethesda System for Reporting Thyroid Cytopathology*, DOI 10.1007/ 978-0-387-87666-5_5,
© Springer Science+Business Media, LLC 2010

practice might be solved one day by the discovery of biomarkers specific for follicular carcinoma.

The goal of this category is to identify all potential follicular carcinomas and refer them for a diagnostic lobectomy. It is not the goal of FNA to identify all follicular neoplasms, because adenomas are clinically innocuous, and there is little if any evidence to suggest progression from adenoma to carcinoma in the thyroid. Nevertheless, the terms FN and SFN are preferred over "suspicious for follicular carcinoma" for several reasons. Both FN and SFN have an established tradition in many laboratories; the terms recognize the impossibility of distinguishing adenoma from carcinoma by FNA; and both terms recognize that the majority of cases interpreted as FN/SFN turn out to be follicular adenomas simply because follicular adenomas outnumber follicular carcinomas in the population.

It is important to point out that cytologic-histologic correlation for the follicular-patterned thyroid nodules is hindered somewhat by the imperfect reproducibility among histopathologists in the diagnosis of nodular hyperplasia, follicular adenoma, follicular carcinoma, and the follicular variant of papillary carcinoma.[13]

Definition

The general diagnostic category "Follicular neoplasm" or "Suspicious for a follicular neoplasm" refers to a cellular aspirate comprised of follicular cells, most of which are arranged in an altered architectural pattern characterized by significant cell crowding and/or microfollicle formation. Cases that demonstrate the nuclear features of papillary carcinoma are excluded from this category.

Criteria

Cytologic preparations are moderately or markedly cellular (Figs. 5.1 a, b).

There is a significant alteration in the follicular cell architecture, characterized by cell crowding, microfollicles, and dispersed isolated cells (Figs. 5.2 a, b).

Follicular cells are normal-sized or enlarged and relatively uniform, with scant or moderate amounts of cytoplasm.

Nuclei are round and slightly hyperchromatic, with inconspicuous nucleoli (Figs. 5.2 a, b).

Some nuclear atypia may be seen, with enlarged, variably sized nuclei and prominent nucleoli (Figs. 5.3 a, b).

Colloid is scant or absent.

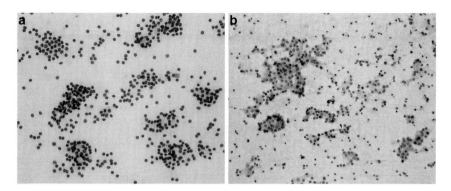

Figure 5.1. (**a, b**) Follicular neoplasm/Suspicious for a follicular neoplasm. Low power shows a highly cellular aspirate composed of uniform follicular cells arranged in crowded clusters and microfollicles (**a**: smear, Diff-Quik stain; b: smear, Papanicolaou stain).

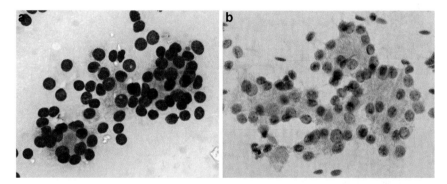

Figure 5.2. (**a**) Follicular neoplasm/Suspicious for a follicular neoplasm. The crowded follicular cells have round nuclei of similar size and faint cytoplasm (smear, Diff-Quik stain). (**b**) Follicular neoplasm/Suspicious for a follicular neoplasm. Follicular cells are arranged as microfollicles and have round nuclei, evenly dispersed, granular chromatin, and small nucleoli (smear, Papanicolaou stain).

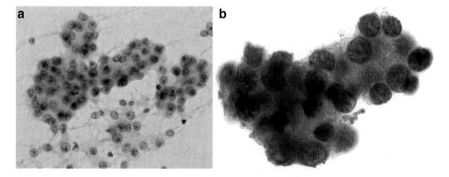

Figure 5.3. (**a, b**): Follicular neoplasm/Suspicious for a follicular neoplasm. Follicular cells in crowded, microfollicular arrangements show slight size variation, chromatin that is more "open" (less granular), and enlarged nucleoli (**a**: smear, Papanicolaou stain; **b**: ThinPrep, Papanicolaou stain).

Explanatory Notes

The hallmark of the FN/SFN specimen is the presence of a significant architectural alteration in the majority the follicular cells. The altered architecture takes the form of crowded and overlapping follicular cells (Figs. 5.4 a, b), some or most of which are arranged as microfollicles. To improve reproducibility, it has been proposed that the "microfollicle" designation must be limited to crowded, flat groups of less than 15 follicular cells arranged in a circle that is at least two-thirds complete,[14] but this recommendation has not been tested in a prospective study. A small amount of inspissated colloid may be present within the microfollicle (Figs. 5.5 a, b). Microfollicles tend to be relatively uniform in size ("equisized"). In some cases, crowded follicular cells form ribbons of overlapping cells ("trabeculae") that are more prominent than the microfollicles (Fig. 5.6).

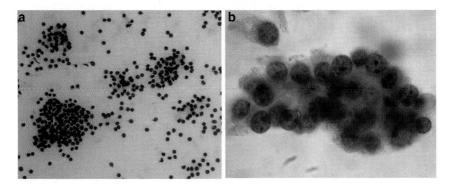

Figure 5.4. (**a, b**) Follicular neoplasm/Suspicious for a follicular neoplasm. Microfollicles demonstrate nuclear overlap. Some are loosely cohesive clusters, and there are dispersed isolated cells (**a**: smear, Diff-Quik stain; **b**: ThinPrep, Papanicolaou stain).

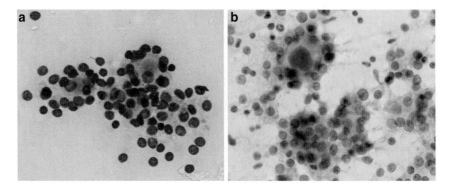

Figure 5.5. (**a, b**) Follicular neoplasm/Suspicious for a follicular neoplasm. Microfollicles may contain small amounts of colloid. (**a**: smear, Diff-Quik stain; **b**: smear, Papanicolaou stain).

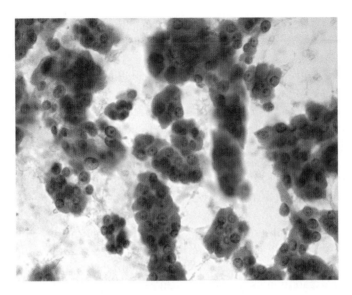

Figure 5.6. Follicular neoplasm/Suspicious for a follicular neoplasm. In some cases, trabeculae of crowded follicular cells are more conspicuous than microfollicles (smear, Papanicolaou stain).

It is important to recognize that rare macrofollicle fragments as well as some background colloid may be present in FN/SFN specimens. A small fragment of follicular cells is not necessarily a microfollicle: an important defining feature of the microfollicle is the crowding and overlapping of the follicular cells.

Cystic change is not common unless the neoplasm is large, at which point it may undergo central degenerative change with associated findings (foamy and hemosiderin-laden macrophages).

Although most FN/SFNs are highly cellular specimens, cellularity by itself is not sufficient to merit this designation.[15] If the majority of follicular cells are arranged in macrofollicle fragments (variably sized fragments without overlap or crowding), the sample can be considered benign. Similarly, nuclear atypia by itself is not diagnostic of malignancy or even neoplasia, as hyperplastic nodules and follicular adenomas can demonstrate nuclear enlargement and hyperchromasia.[16–18]

An occasional dilemma is the sparsely cellular sample composed predominantly of microfollicles. Most cytologists are reluctant to make an FN/SFN interpretation on a sparsely cellular sample because of the discrepancy between the cellularity and the cell pattern. It is reasonable to interpret such cases as ATYPIA OF UNDETERMINED SIGNIFICANCE (see Chap. 4). In such cases, a repeat aspiration is a reasonable approach and is likely to resolve the discrepancy.

If the follicular cells show features of papillary thyroid carcinoma, the specimen should not be interpreted as FN/SFN but rather as "MALIGNANT, Papillary thyroid carcinoma" or "SUSPICIOUS FOR MALIGNANCY, suspicious for papillary thyroid carcinoma," depending on the quality and quantity of the cytologic changes.

Fine needle aspirations of parathyroid adenomas are composed of cells that resemble crowded and overlapping follicular cells (Fig. 5.7). Even when the FNA is performed with ultrasound guidance, it may not be clear to the aspirator that the lesion arises from a parathyroid gland rather than the thyroid. When submitted as a "thyroid FNA" specimen, parathyroid adenomas are often misinterpreted as FN/SFN.

There are robust data on the predictive value of the FN/SFN interpretation because most patients with this FNA result undergo surgery.[3,4,9,11] The likelihood that the nodule is neoplastic is 65–85%. The rate of malignancy is significantly lower, at 12–32%. Moreover, not all the malignancies prove to be follicular carcinomas: many if not most of the malignancies (27–68%) are interpreted histologically as papillary thyroid carcinoma.[3,4,9,11] There are a number of explanations for this discrepancy. Some tumors may have subtle features of papillary carcinoma that were not appreciated on the FNA sample. In other cases, however, the discrepancy may be due to the imperfect reproducibility of the histologic diagnoses of follicular carcinoma and follicular variant of papillary carcinoma.[13]

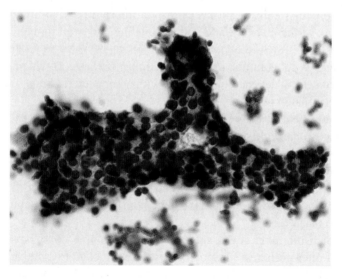

FIGURE 5.7. Follicular neoplasm/Suspicious for a follicular neoplasm. These crowded, uniform cells are arranged in thick trabeculae mimicking neoplastic follicular cells. Lobectomy revealed an unsuspected parathyroid adenoma (smear, hematoxylin and eosin stain).

Management

The recommended management of a patient with a diagnosis of FN/SFN is surgical excision of the lesion, most often a hemithyroidectomy or lobectomy.[19-21]

Sample Reports

If an aspirate is interpreted as FN/SFN, it is implied that the sample is adequate for evaluation. (An explicit statement of adequacy is optional.) The general category FN/SFN is a self-sufficient interpretation; narrative comments that follow are optional. An educational note specifying the risk of malignancy for this interpretation, derived from the laboratory itself or from the literature, is optional. For the FN/SFN category, the risk of malignancy is 12–32%.[3,4,9,11]

Example 1:
SUSPICIOUS FOR A FOLLICULAR NEOPLASM.

Example 2:
FOLLICULAR NEOPLASM.

Example 3:
SUSPICIOUS FOR A FOLLICULAR NEOPLASM.
Cellular aspirate of follicular cells with a predominantly microfollicular architecture, scattered isolated cells, and scant colloid.

Example 4:
SUSPICIOUS FOR A FOLLICULAR NEOPLASM.
Cellular aspirate composed predominantly of crowded uniform cells without colloid. The features suggest a follicular neoplasm, but the possibility of a parathyroid lesion cannot be excluded. Correlation with clinical, serologic, and radiologic findings should be considered.

References

1. Baloch ZW, LiVolsi VA, Asa SL, et al. Diagnostic terminology and morphologic criteria for cytologic diagnosis of thyroid lesions: a synopsis of the National Cancer Institute Thyroid Fine-Needle Aspiration State of the Science Conference. *Diagn Cytopathol.* 2008;36(6):425-37.
2. Gharib H, Goellner JR. Fine-needle aspiration biopsy of the thyroid: an appraisal. *Ann Int Med.* 1993;118:282-9.
3. Yang J, Schnadig V, Logrono R, Wasserman PG. Fine-needle aspiration of thyroid nodules: a study of 4703 patients with histologic and clinical correlations. *Cancer.* 2007;111(5): 306-15.

4. Deveci MS, Deveci G, LiVolsi VA, Baloch ZW. Fine-needle aspiration of follicular lesions of the thyroid Diagnosis and follow-Up. *Cytojournal*. 2006;3:9.

5. Baloch ZW, Fleisher S, LiVolsi VA, Gupta PK. Diagnosis of "follicular neoplasm": a gray zone in thyroid fine-needle aspiration cytology. *Diagn Cytopathol*. 2002;26(1):41-4.

6. Yang GC, Liebeskind D, Messina AV. Should cytopathologists stop reporting follicular neoplasms on fine-needle aspiration of the thyroid? *Cancer*. 2003;99(2):69-74.

7. Greaves TS, Olvera M, Florentine BD, et al. Follicular lesions of thyroid: a 5-year fine-needle aspiration experience. *Cancer*. 2000;90(6):335-41.

8. Guidelines of the Papanicolaou Society of Cytopathology for the examination of fine-needle aspiration specimens from thyroid nodules. The Papanicolaou Society of Cytopathology Task Force on Standards of Practice. *Diagn Cytopathol* 1996;15(1):84-9.

9. Yassa L, Cibas ES, Benson CB, et al. Long-term assessment of a multidisciplinary approach to thyroid nodule diagnostic evaluation. *Cancer*. 2007;111(6):508-16.

10. Wang HH. Reporting thyroid fine-needle aspiration: literature review and a proposal. *Diagn Cytopathol*. 2006;34(1):67-76.

11. Schlinkert RT, van Heerden JA, Goellner JR, et al. Factors that predict malignant thyroid lesions when fine-needle aspiration is "suspicious for follicular neoplasm". *Mayo Clin Proc*. 1997;72(10):913-6.

12. Kelman AS, Rathan A, Leibowitz J, Burstein DE, Haber RS. Thyroid cytology and the risk of malignancy in thyroid nodules: importance of nuclear atypia in indeterminate specimens. *Thyroid*. 2001;11(3):271-7.

13. Elsheikh TM, Asa SL, Chan JK, et al. Interobserver and intraobserver variation among experts in the diagnosis of thyroid follicular lesions with borderline nuclear features of papillary carcinoma. *Am J Clin Pathol*. 2008;130(5):736-44.

14. Renshaw AA, Wang E, Wilbur D, Hughes JH, Haja J, Henry MR. Interobserver agreement on microfollicles in thyroid fine-needle aspirates. *Arch Pathol Lab Med*. 2006;130(2):148-52.

15. Suen KC. How does one separate cellular follicular lesions of the thyroid by fine-needle aspiration biopsy? *Diagn Cytopathol*. 1988;4:78-81.

16. Stelow EB, Bardales RH, Crary GS, et al. Interobserver variability in thyroid fine-needle aspiration interpretation of lesions showing predominantly colloid and follicular groups. *Am J Clin Pathol*. 2005;124(2):239-44.

17. Clary KM, Condel JL, Liu Y, Johnson DR, Grzybicki DM, Raab SS. Interobserver variability in the fine needle aspiration biopsy diagnosis of follicular lesions of the thyroid gland. *Acta Cytol*. 2005;49(4):378-82.

18. Goldstein RE, Netterville JL, Burkey B, Johnson JE. Implications of follicular neoplasms, atypia, and lesions suspicious for malignancy diagnosed by fine-needle aspiration of thyroid nodules. *Ann Surg* 2002;235(5):656–662; discussion 62-4.

19. Layfield LJ, Abrams J, Cochand-Priollet B, et al. Post-thyroid FNA testing and treatment options: a synopsis of the National Cancer Institute Thyroid Fine Needle Aspiration State of the Science Conference. *Diagn Cytopathol*. 2008;36(6):442-8.

20. Cooper DS, Doherty GM, Haugen BR, et al. Management guidelines for patients with thyroid nodules and differentiated thyroid cancer. *Thyroid*. 2006;16(2):109-42.

21. Gharib H, Papini E, Valcavi R. et al. American Association of Clinical Endocrinologists and Associazione Medici Endocrinologi medical guidelines for clinical practice for the diagnosis and management of thyroid nodules. *Endocr Pract* 2006;12(1):63-102.

Chapter 6

Follicular Neoplasm, Hürthle Cell Type/Suspicious for a Follicular Neoplasm, Hürthle Cell Type

William C. Faquin, Claire W. Michael, Andrew A. Renshaw, and Philippe Vielh

Background

Ewing coined the term "Hürthle cell" in 1928 based upon the description of a cell made by Hürthle in 1894. The term has become entrenched in the thyroid lexicon, even though Hürthle's original description is now believed to represent a parafollicular or C-cell of the thyroid gland.[1] In 1898, Askanazy was the first to describe the follicular-derived Hürthle cell as we know it today.[2] The Hürthle cell (also called Askanazy cell, oxyphilic cell, and oncocyte) is defined morphologically as a thyroid follicular cell with an abundance of finely granular cytoplasm. Most Hürthle cells have an enlarged, round to oval nucleus, and some have a prominent nucleolus.

Hürthle cells are commonly seen in reactive/hyperplastic conditions like lymphocytic (Hashimoto's) thyroiditis (LT) and multinodular goiter (MNG), where they are considered metaplastic, non-neoplastic follicular cells, but they can also be neoplastic (Hürthle cell adenoma and Hürthle cell carcinoma). The World Health Organization (WHO) considers Hürthle cell adenoma and carcinoma as variants of follicular adenoma and carcinoma.[3] In the Bethesda System for reporting thyroid FNA results, FNA specimens that are suspicious for a Hürthle cell neoplasm are distinguished from those suspicious for a follicular neoplasm for two reasons: (1) there is a striking morphologic difference between these two cytologic patterns, which raises different diagnostic considerations, and (2) there are emerging data to suggest that follicular and Hürthle cell carcinomas may be genetically different neoplasms.[4] For example, the PAX8-PPARγ rearrangement is seen in 26–53% of follicular carcinomas but virtually never in Hürthle cell carcinomas.[5,6]

In the Bethesda System, the terms "Follicular neoplasm, Hürthle cell type" and "Suspicious for a follicular neoplasm, Hürthle cell type" are

Syed Z. Ali and Edmund S. Cibas (eds.), *The Bethesda System for Reporting Thyroid Cytopathology*, DOI 10.1007/ 978-0-387-87666-5_6,
© Springer Science+Business Media, LLC 2010

equally acceptable for this category (see Sample Reports at the end of this chapter). "Suspicious for a follicular neoplasm, Hürthle cell type (SFNHCT)" is preferred over "Follicular neoplasm, Hürthle cell type (FNHCT)" by some laboratories because a significant proportion of cases (16–25%) prove not to be neoplasms but rather hyperplastic proliferations of Hürthle cells in nodular goiter or LT.[7,8]

Hürthle cell carcinomas are uncommon, representing only 15–20% of all follicular carcinomas.[9] As with (non-oncocytic) follicular adenoma and carcinoma, the distinction between Hürthle cell adenoma and carcinoma is based upon histologic evidence of transcapsular and/or vascular invasion. For this reason, thyroid FNA is used as a screening test for the detection of a probable Hürthle cell neoplasm that requires surgical excision for precise histologic classification.[10] Although FNA is highly sensitive for detecting Hürthle cell carcinomas, its specificity is low: most nodules diagnosed by FNA as FNHCT/SFNHCT are benign[7,8,11–13] because Hürthle cell adenomas outnumber carcinomas. Currently, no ancillary techniques can reliably distinguish between a Hürthle cell adenoma and carcinoma.

Definition

The interpretation "Follicular neoplasm, Hurthle cell type" or "Suspicious for a follicular neoplasm, Hürthle cell type" refers to a cellular aspirate that consists exclusively (or almost exclusively) of Hürthle cells. Oncocytic cells with nuclear features of papillary carcinoma are excluded from this category.

Criteria

Specimens are moderately to markedly cellular (Fig. 6.1).

The sample consists exclusively (or almost exclusively) of **Hürthle cells** (Fig. 6.2):

- abundant finely granular cytoplasm (blue or grey-pink with Romanowsky stains, green with Papanicolaou, pink with hematoxylin and eosin)
- enlarged, central or eccentrically located, round nucleus
- prominent nucleolus
- small cells with high nuclear/cytoplasmic (N/C) ratio (small cell dysplasia) (Figs. 6.3–6.4)
- large cells with at least 2x variability in nuclear size (large cell dysplasia) (Fig. 6.5)

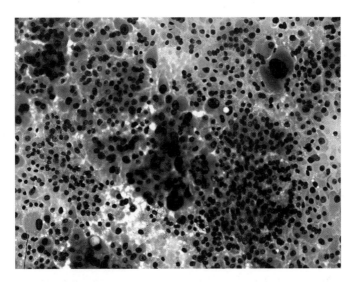

Figure 6.1. Follicular neoplasm, Hürthle cell type/Suspicious for a follicular neoplasm, Hürthle cell type. The aspirate is very cellular and consists of Hürthle cells of variable size arranged as isolated cells and in crowded groups; colloid is absent (smear, Diff-Quik stain).

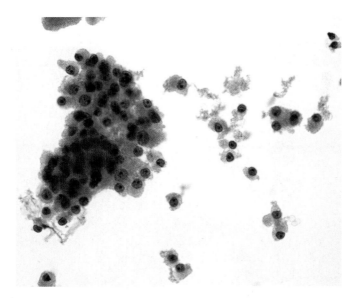

Figure 6.2. Follicular neoplasm, Hürthle cell type/Suspicious for a follicular neoplasm, Hürthle cell type. The aspirate consists of a pure population of Hürthle cells in small crowded groups and as isolated cells in a background that lacks colloid and lymphocytes (ThinPrep, Papanicolaou stain).

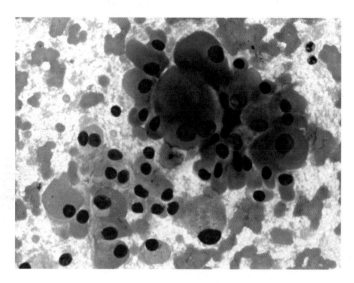

FIGURE 6.3. Follicular neoplasm, Hürthle cell type/Suspicious for a follicular neoplasm, Hürthle cell type. The aspirate consists of a population of loosely cohesive Hürthle cells. The cells are highly variable in size and amount of cytoplasm, transitioning from gigantic cells with abundant cytoplasm and macronucleoli to smaller, uniform Hürthle cells with a high nuclear/cytoplasmic (N/C) ratio (smear, Diff-Quik stain).

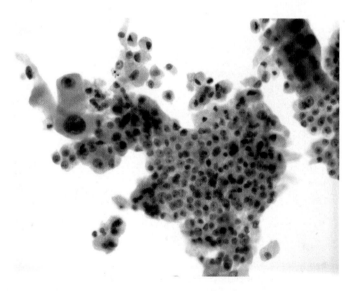

FIGURE 6.4. Follicular neoplasm, Hürthle cell type/Suspicious for a follicular neoplasm, Hürthle cell type. This cellular aspirate consists exclusively of Hürthle cells arranged in syncytial-like sheets and as isolated cells. The cells exhibit marked variation in cell and nuclear size (mixed small and large cell dysplasia) (ThinPrep, Papanicolaou stain).

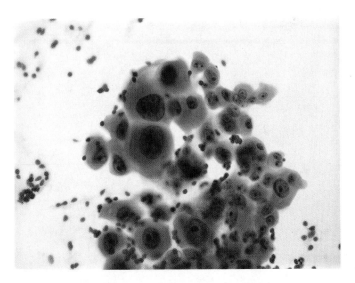

FIGURE 6.5. Follicular neoplasm, Hürthle cell type/Suspicious for a follicular neoplasm, Hürthle cell type. This cellular aspirate consists of loosely cohesive, markedly enlarged Hürthle cells with marked anisonucleosis and macronucleoli (large cell dysplasia) (smear, Papanicolaou stain).

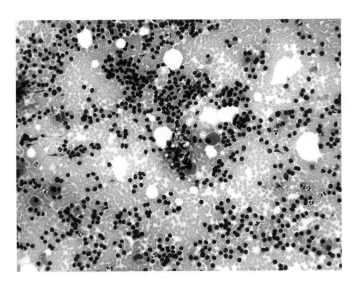

FIGURE 6.6. Follicular neoplasm, Hürthle cell type/Suspicious for a follicular neoplasm, Hürthle cell type. The aspirate is cellular and consists exclusively of Hürthle cells in an isolated-cell pattern (smear, Diff-Quik stain).

The Hürthle cells are dispersed predominantly as isolated cells (Fig. 6.6), but sometimes arranged in crowded, syncytial-like arrangements (Fig. 6.4). There is usually little or no colloid.

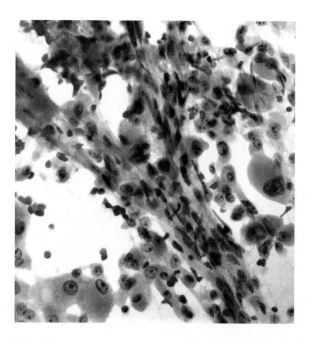

Figure 6.7. Follicular neoplasm, Hürthle cell type/Suspicious for a follicular neoplasm, Hürthle cell type. A cellular aspirate consists of noncohesive Hürthle cells with both large and small cell dysplasia. Colloid is absent, and a small transgressing vessel is present in the center (smear, Papanicolaou stain).

There are virtually no lymphocytes (excluding blood elements) or plasma cells.

Transgressing vessels are present in some cases (Fig. 6.7).

Explanatory Notes

The typical FNHCT/SFNHCT aspirate is very cellular and composed exclusively of Hürthle cells (excluding blood elements).[4,14,15] A small number of benign follicular cells may be present, but this is exceptional. In most cases, the Hürthle cells are dispersed predominantly as isolated cells.[16,17] They can be very large cells with large amounts of granular cytoplasm ("large cell dysplasia") or relatively small Hürthle cells ("small cell dysplasia").[16,18] Admixtures of small and large Hürthle cells are seen in some cases. Anisonucleosis and hyperchromasia are seen in some cases, but nuclear atypia by itself is an unreliable feature for the diagnosis – in fact, very marked hyperchromasia, anisonucleosis, and nuclear membrane irregularity of Hürthle cells can be seen in MNG and LT.[4] Colloid is usually scant or absent.[17]

When an aspirate has all (or most) of the aforementioned features, the diagnosis of FNHCT/SFNHCT is straightforward. Problems arise with regard to 1. the minimum necessary criteria for the diagnosis, 2. the best way to handle Hürthle cell proliferations in a patient with MNG or LT, and 3. the distinction from papillary carcinoma, medullary carcinoma, and parathyroid tumors.

With regard to the minimum criteria for diagnosing FNHCT/SFNHCT, there are three general problematic scenarios: the sparsely cellular specimen composed entirely of Hürthle cells; the moderately-to-markedly cellular specimen composed exclusively of Hürthle cells (or "Hürthle-oid" cells) without atypia; and the clearly abnormal specimen with partial or minimal Hürthle cell differentiation. A sparsely cellular aspirate does not preclude a Hürthle cell carcinoma.[18] Most cytopathologists, however, are reluctant to make the diagnosis of FNHCT/SFNHCT on a scant aspirate, and, as a result, these aspirates are usually diagnosed as "Atypia of Undetermined Significance (AUS)" (see Chapter 4). A reaspiration can often resolve the diagnostic difficulty. The moderately-to-markedly cellular aspirate composed entirely of nonatypical Hürthle cells is more controversial. If abundant colloid accompanies a pure population of Hürthle cells, it is a common practice to interpret the sample as benign. In the absence of abundant colloid, there are two different approaches to the cellular aspirate composed entirely of Hürthle cells without atypia. Many cytopathologists diagnose such cases as FNHCT/SFNHCT. Two groups of investigators have recently shown, however, that Hürthle cell aspirates that have neither small-cell nor large-cell dysplasia are almost never malignant.[16,18] As a result, some cytopathologists diagnose pure Hürthle cell cases without atypia (i.e., dysplasia) as benign, accompanied by an optional note like the following: "Although the predominance of Hürthle cells raises the possibility of a Hürthle cell neoplasm, the absence of atypia suggests that it is benign." Typically, such patients are followed clinically with periodic physical and sonographic examinations. Similarly, it is not uncommon to encounter a relatively bland aspirate composed of cells with minimal atypia but "Hürthle-oid" features with more granular cytoplasm than is seen in typical follicular cells but not as much as is seen in usual Hürthle cells. Most of these cases can also be diagnosed as benign with a similar (optional) note ("the findings raise the possibility of a Hürthle cell neoplasm, but the lack of atypia suggests it is benign"). Finally, there are clearly abnormal cases (markedly cellular specimens with crowding and overlapping of cells, etc.) where Hürthle cell differentiation is focal rather than diffuse, or not as well developed as in most HCNs. In such cases, the diagnostic choices are "Follicular Neoplasm/Suspicious for a Follicular Neoplasm" versus FNHCT/SFNHCT. When Hürthle cell differentiation is clear cut but only focal, it is advisable to follow the guidelines of the WHO, which considers only those follicular neoplasms that are comprised of >75% Hürthle cells to be a HCNs.[3] Thus, a suspicious FNA in which <75% of the abnormal cells are well-developed Hürthle cells should be diagnosed as "Follicular Neoplasm/Suspicious for a Follicular Neoplasm" rather than FNHCT/SFNHCT. When Hürthle cell differentiation is not clear cut (more granular cytoplasm than normal follicular cells, but not as much as usual Hürthle cells), it is often impossible to make a definitive distinction between follicular and Hürthle cell differentiation. Because the usual management is the same for both entities, a practical solution is to diagnose these aspirates as "Follicular Neoplasm/Suspicious for a Follicular Neoplasm," with the comment "Some Hürthle cell differentiation is present, and therefore a Hürthle cell neoplasm cannot be ruled out."

The classic FNHCT/SFNHCT pattern can be mimicked by a variety of other conditions, particularly MNG with focal Hürthle cell change and LT with Hürthle cell hyperplasia. Prominent Hürthle cell metaplasia often accompanies MNG. Typically one sees a mixture of elements: flat, cohesive sheets of Hürthle cells admixed with normal follicular cells and a moderate to abundant amount of colloid (Fig. 6.8). Aspirates with these features are easily recognized as benign and should not be interpreted as FNHCT/SFNHCT. Thus, whereas, most aspirates of HCNs consist of a pure population of Hürthle cells, a mixture of Hürthle cells and non-oncocytic follicular

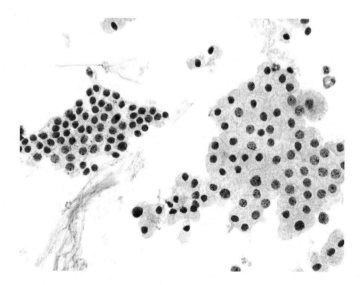

Figure 6.8. Benign (multinodular hyperplasia with a prominent Hürthle cell component). There are benign follicular cells (*left*) and Hürthle cells (*right*) in cohesive flat sheets, with a moderate amount of "tissue-paper" colloid. Such cases should not be called "Follicular neoplasm, Hürthle cell type/Suspicious for a follicular neoplasm, Hürthle cell type" (ThinPrep, Papanicolaou stain).

cells is more indicative of a hyperplastic nodule. Exceptions to this rule occur and represent a limitation in the precise classification of these lesions by FNA. It is possible, for example, to aspirate normal follicular cells from adjacent thyroid tissue when aspirating a HCN, particularly if the FNA is done without ultrasound guidance. Thus, a minor component of normal follicular cells does not exclude an HCN. Conversely, some nodules in patients with MNG are composed exclusively of Hürthle cells (with or without significant nuclear atypia); such benign hyperplastic nodules masquerade as an HCN. Clinical-cytologic correlation is a reasonable approach in such cases and can be performed by either the cytopathologist or the clinician. For example, in a patient known to have multiple nodules, it is acceptable to diagnose an exclusively Hürthle cell specimen as either FNHCT/SFNHCT or as AUS. If interpreted as AUS, an explanatory note that raises the possibility of a Hürthle cell hyperplasia can be very helpful (see Chapter 4, Sample Report Example 6). The note that accompanies the interpretation in this setting is meant to more accurately reflect the underlying risk of malignancy, which, although not well characterized, is considered to be lower than for FNHCT/SFNHCT in general. The goal is to provide the clinician with the opportunity to avoid an unnecessary lobectomy in some of these patients. Note that in this setting, the usual management of a patient with an AUS result - a repeat aspiration - is unlikely to add any helpful information.

In most nodules from patients with LT, lymphocytes predominate over Hürthle cells, and the benign aspirate is easily distinguished from an HCN on this basis. In some patients with LT, however, Hürthle cell proliferation can produce nodules that exceed 1cm in diameter and are composed of Hürthle cells with little or no lymphoid infiltrate (Fig. 6.9).[19] When the lymphoid component is absent or inconspicuous, it can be difficult to exclude an HCN. There may be a clue to the correct interpretation: in LT nodules, the Hürthle cells are "atypical" in a stereotypical way: they form small cohesive clusters of 3–10 cells containing large nuclei and smudgy, sometimes glassy chromatin. This nuclear atypia can mimic that found in papillary carcinoma, but it is not typical of HCNs.

Knowing that a patient has LT may impact the interpretation. In a patient known to have LT, it is acceptable to diagnose an exclusively (or virtually exclusively) Hürthle cell specimen as either FNHCT/SFNHCT or AUS. If interpreted as AUS, a note explaining that a benign Hürthle cell hyperplasia is favored can be very helpful (see Chapter 4, see Sample Report Example 7). As in patients with MNG, the note that accompanies the AUS interpretation in a patient with LT is meant to more accurately reflect the underlying risk of malignancy, which, although not well characterized, is considered to be lower than for FNHCT/SFNHCT in general. The goal is to provide the clinician with the opportunity to avoid an unnecessary lobectomy in some of

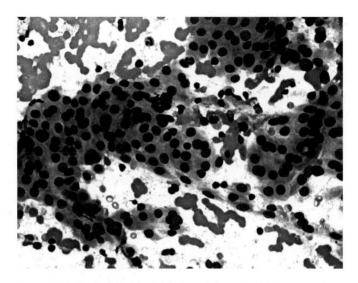

FIGURE 6.9. Atypia of undetermined significance (AUS). This oncocytic nodule in a patient with lymphocytic (Hashimoto's) thyroiditis exhibits a predominance of Hürthle cells in crowded groups with very few lymphocytes. In a patient with a known clinical diagnosis of lymphocytic (Hashimoto's) thyroiditis, such cases can be interpreted as AUS (smear, Diff-Quik stain).

these patients. Note that in this setting, the usual management for an AUS diagnosis - a repeat aspiration - is unlikely to provide any helpful information. The AUS interpretation in this setting does not ask for a repeat aspiration, but rather encourages clinical-cytologic correlation to more accurately predict the risk of malignancy.

The differential diagnosis of FNHCT/SFNHCT includes other neoplasms. HCNs can exhibit some of the architectural and nuclear features of papillary carcinoma, including micropapillary groups (Fig. 6.10), fibrovascular cores, pale chromatin, grooves, and intranuclear inclusions, as well as occasional psammoma body-like concretions[3] (Fig. 6.11). Conversely, the cells of many classic papillary carcinomas often show focal oncocytic differentiation. This is particularly extensive in the oncocytic variant of papillary carcinoma (see Chapter 8). The abundance of granular cytoplasm in these neoplasms mimics that of a HCN. Attention to nuclear details usually permits a distinction, but in some cases it may not be possible to determine with certainty whether an aspirate is best classified as a papillary carcinoma or FNHCT/SFNHCT. Such aspirates can be diagnosed either as FNHCT/SFNHCT or "Suspicious for malignancy," accompanied by an explanatory note that includes the differential diagnosis of papillary carcinoma and an HCN. Many of these borderline lesions can be accurately diagnosed at the time of frozen section based on architectural features, thus patients with this diagnosis are candidates

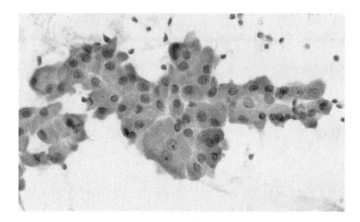

FIGURE 6.10. Follicular neoplasm, Hürthle cell type/Suspicious for a follicular neoplasm, Hürthle cell type. Histologic examination revealed a Hürthle cell carcinoma with papillary features. A subset of Hürthle cell neoplasms exhibits papillary cytoarchitecture, with ocasional cells that have an oval, pale, and grooved nucleus. Such cases can be difficult to distinguish from a papillary thyroid carcinoma (smear, Papanicolaou stain).

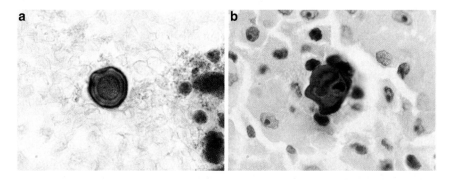

FIGURE 6.11. (**a, b**) Follicular neoplasm, Hürthle cell type/Suspicious for a follicular neoplasm, Hürthle cell type. A minority of Hürthle cell neoplasms contain concentrically laminated concretions that are indistinguishable from psammoma bodies. The correct diagnosis depends on the accompanying cellular features. [(**a**) FNA smear, Papanicolaou stain. (**b**) Subsequent histologic specimen of a Hürthle cell adenoma].

for lobectomy with frozen section and possible completion thyroidectomy at a single surgical procedure.

Some of the characteristic features of HCNs overlap with those of a medullary carcinoma (Fig. 6.12). Many medullary carcinomas are comprised of isolated cells with abundant granular cytoplasm. The prominent nucleolus of most HCNs is absent from most medullary carcinoma cells. With Romanowsky stains, the cytoplasmic granules of Hürthle cells are blue,

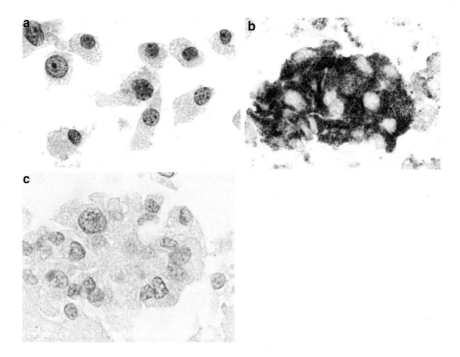

Figure 6.12. (a–c) Follicular neoplasm, Hürthle cell type/Suspicious for a follicular neoplasm, Hürthle cell type. (a) Some Hürthle cell neoplasms can be difficult to distinguish from a medullary carcinoma by cytomorphology alone. This case demonstrates a population of cells with abundant cytoplasm and occasional eccentrically placed nuclei (ThinPrep, Papanicolaou stain). (b) Immunohistochemical studies on a cell block preparation are positive for thyroglobulin. (c) The suspicious cells are negative for calcitonin.

whereas those of medullary carcinoma are usually red. Immunohistochemistry is especially useful in the distinction between Hürthle cells and medullary carcinoma: HCNs are positive for thyroglobulin and negative for calcitonin, whereas medullary carcinomas are negative for thyroglobulin but positive for calcitonin and chromogranin. When employing immunostains, a panel of immunohistochemical stains, including some that are expected to be positive (e.g., thyroglobulin) and others expected to be negative (e.g., calcitonin), is preferable to solitary antibody staining, because aberrant results can occur with any given antibody.

Parathyroid adenomas usually mimic a follicular neoplasm, but some have abundant granular cytoplasm and mimic instead an HCN. Sometimes the radiologist will consider a parathyroid tumor based on imaging characteristics, and occasionally there will be serologic testing results to raise this possibility. In many cases, however, a parathyroid tumor will not be suspected clinically, and the possibility of a parathyroid tumor will need to be raised based on morphologic evaluation of the FNA specimen. In contrast to

HCNs, the cells of a parathyroid adenoma with abundant granular cytoplasm are monomorphous, with round nuclei and "salt and pepper" chromatin. Parathyroid tumors are immunoreactive for chromogranin, synaptophysin, and parathyroid hormone (PTH) and are negative for thyroglobulin and TTF-1. HCNs, by contrast, have more finely textured chromatin, more anisonucleosis, and more highly irregular nuclei; they are immunoreactive for TTF-1 and thyroglobulin. If cyst fluid is obtained and submitted for chemical analysis, a high PTH level can be diagnostically helpful.[20] A conclusive distinction will not always be possible, especially if immunohistochemistry is not available or is inconclusive. In such cases, the possibility of a parathyroid tumor can be raised in the note that accompanies the interpretation.

Sample Reports

If an aspirate is interpreted as FNHCT/SFNHCT, it is implied that the sample is adequate for evaluation. (An explicit statement of adequacy is optional.) The interpretation FNHCT/SFNHCT is self-sufficient; narrative comments that follow are optional.

Example 1:
SUSPICIOUS FOR A FOLLICULAR NEOPLASM, HÜRTHLE CELL TYPE.

Example 2:
FOLLICULAR NEOPLASM, HÜRTHLE CELL TYPE.

Example 3:
SUSPICIOUS FOR A HÜRTHLE CELL NEOPLASM.
Cellular aspirate consisting predominantly of Hürthle cells in syncytial-like sheets and crowded clusters.

Example 4:
HÜRTHLE CELL NEOPLASM.
Cellular aspirate consisting of abundant isolated Hürthle cells in the absence of colloid.

Example 5:
SUSPICIOUS FOR A HÜRTHLE CELL NEOPLASM.
Cellular aspirate of follicular cells with oncocytic features, including occasional nuclear grooves and focal papillary architecture. The findings raise the possibility of a Hürthle cell neoplasm with papillary features, but a papillary thyroid carcinoma cannot be excluded.

Example 6:
SUSPICIOUS FOR A HÜRTHLE CELL NEOPLASM.

Cellular aspirate composed of cells with abundant granular cytoplasm. The findings raise the possibility of a Hürthle cell neoplasm, but a parathyroid tumor cannot be excluded. Correlation with clinical findings, imaging findings, and serologic testing results might be helpful.

References

1. Hurthle K. A study of the secretory process of the thyroid gland. *Arch F D Ges Physiol*. 1894:56.
2. Askanazy M. Pathologisch-anatomische beitrage zure kenntnis des morbus basedowii, insbesondere uber die dabei auftretende muskelergrankung. *Dtsch Arch Klin Med*. 1898;61:118.
3. DeLellis RA, Lloyd RV, Heitz PU, Eng C, eds. *World Health Organization Classification of Tumours. Pathology and Genetics of Tumours of Endocrine Organs*. Lyon: IARC Press; 2004.
4. Baloch ZW, LiVolsi VA, Asa SL, et al. Diagnostic terminology and morphologic criteria for cytologic diagnosis of thyroid lesions: a synopsis of the National Cancer Institute Thyroid Fine-Needle Aspiration State of the Science Conference. *Diagn Cytopathol*. 2008;36(6):425-437.
5. French CA, Alexander EK, Cibas ES, et al. Genetic and biological subgroups of low-stage follicular thyroid cancer. *Am J Pathol*. 2003;162(4):1053-1060.
6. Nikiforova MN, Biddinger PW, Caudill CM, et al. PAX8-PPARgamma rearrangement in thyroid tumors: RT-PCR and immunohistochemical analyses. *Am J Surg Pathol*. 2002;26(8):1016-1023.
7. Giorgadze T, Rossi ED, Fadda G, et al. Does the fine-needle aspiration diagnosis of "Hurthle-cell neoplasm/follicular neoplasm with oncocytic features" denote increased risk of malignancy? *Diagn Cytopathol*. 2004;31(5):307-312.
8. Pu RT, Yang J, Wasserman PG, et al. Does Hurthle cell lesion/neoplasm predict malignancy more than follicular lesion/neoplasm on thyroid fine-needle aspiration? *Diagn Cytopathol*. 2006;34(5):330-334.
9. Rosai J, Carcangiu ML, DeLellis RA. *Tumors of the thyroid gland. Atlas of Tumor Pathology Fascicle 5*. 3rd series. Washington, DC: Armed Forces Institute of Pathology; 1992.
10. Clark DP, Faquin WC. *Thyroid Cytopathology*. New York: Springer; 2005:88-102.
11. Renshaw AA. Accuracy of thyroid fine-needle aspiration using receiver operator characteristic curves. *Am J Clin Pathol*. 2001;116:477-482.
12. Amrikachi M, Ramzy I, Rubenfeld S, et al. Accuracy of fine-needle aspiration of thyroid: a review of 6226 cases and correlation with surgical or clinical outcome. *Arch Pathol Lab Med*. 2001;125:484-488.
13. Gharib H, Goellner JR, Johnson DA. Fine-needle aspiration cytology of the thyroid: a 12-year experience with 11, 000 biopsies. *Clin Lab Med*. 1993;13:699-709.
14. Kini SR, Miller JM, Hamburger JI. Cytopathology of Hurthle cell lesions of the thyroid gland by fine needle aspiration. *Acta Cytol*. 1981;25(6):647-652.
15. Nguyen GK, Husain M, Akin MR. Cytodiagnosis of benign and malignant Hurthle cell lesions of the thyroid by fine-needle aspiration biopsy. *Diagn Cytopathol*. 1999;20(5):261-265.
16. Wu HH, Clouse J, Ren R. Fine-needle aspiration cytology of Hurthle cell carcinoma of the thyroid. *Diagn Cytopathol*. 2008;36(3):149-154.

17. Elliott DD, Pitman MB, Bloom L, et al. Fine-needle aspiration biopsy of Hurthle cell lesions of the thyroid gland: a cytomorphologic study of 139 cases with statistical analysis. *Cancer.* 2006;108(2):102-109.
18. Renshaw AA. Hurthle cell carcinoma is a better gold standard than Hurthle cell neoplasm for fine-needle aspiration of the thyroid: defining more consistent and specific cytologic criteria. *Cancer.* 2002;96(5):261-266.
19. Takashima S, Matsuzuka F, Nagareda T, et al. Thyroid nodules associated with Hashimoto thyroiditis: assessment with US. *Radiology.* 1992;185(1):125-130.
20. Owens CL, Rekhtman N, Sokoll L, et al. Parathyroid hormone assay in fine-needle aspirate is useful in differentiating inadvertently sampled parathyroid tissue from thyroid lesions. *Diagn Cytopathol.* 2008;36(4):227-231.

Chapter 7

Suspicious for Malignancy

Helen H. Wang, Armando C. Filie,
Douglas P. Clark, and Celeste N. Powers

Background

Most primary thyroid malignancies have distinctive cytologic features and are easily recognizable on fine needle aspiration (FNA). The exceptions are follicular and Hürthle cell carcinomas (addressed in Chaps. 5 and 6). Although the cytologic features of papillary thyroid carcinoma (PTC), medullary thyroid carcinoma (MTC), and lymphoma are well-established (see Chaps. 8, 9, and 12), in any given specimen they may be quantitatively and/or qualitatively insufficient for a definitive diagnosis. Reasons for diagnostic uncertainty in such cases include suboptimal sampling or preservation, an unusual variant of PTC and MTC, and overlapping cytomorphologic (particularly nuclear) features with other thyroid conditions. The benign follicular cells in some cases of lymphocytic (Hashimoto) thyroiditis (LT) can be difficult to distinguish from those of PTC, and the lymphoid cells of LT can be difficult to distinguish from those of a lymphoma of mucosa-associated lymphoid tissue (MALT lymphoma). A category that conveys a strong suspicion for malignancy, therefore, is a necessity for thyroid FNA, and in the Bethesda System, it is called "Suspicious for Malignancy (SFM)."[1] SFM is a heterogeneous category because it includes a variety of different malignancies. Most SFM cases are suspicious for PTC, although in many published series the type of suspected malignancy is not specified. When specified, the percentage of total thyroid FNA cases that fall into the "suspicious for PTC" category ranges from 2.4% to 7.9%.[2–5] This category should be used judiciously so that patients are managed as appropriately as possible.

The aim of segregating a "suspicious" category apart from a "malignant" category is to preserve the very high positive predictive value (PPV) of the malignant category without compromising the overall sensitivity of the procedure. An SFM interpretation indicates to clinicians the less than definitive nature of the diagnosis and allows for alternative management options

Syed Z. Ali and Edmund S. Cibas (eds.), *The Bethesda System for Reporting Thyroid Cytopathology*, DOI 10.1007/ 978-0-387-87666-5_7,
© Springer Science+Business Media, LLC 2010

(e.g., surgical lobectomy with intra-operative frozen section) before definitive surgery (total thyroidectomy) is performed. A distinction between a malignant and suspicious diagnosis (and between suspicious and atypical) is admittedly subjective. A malignant diagnosis should be reserved for those cases that show sufficient cellularity and most, if not all, of the diagnostic features of an entity. An SFM interpretation is rendered when some of the diagnostic features are either absent or equivocal. The PPV of the SFM category should be greater than 50% and ideally in the range of 65–85%,[6,7] especially at institutions where surgeons are likely to perform a total thyroidectomy based on an SFM interpretation.

Definition

A specimen is suspicious for malignancy (SFM) when some features of malignancy (mainly PTC in this context) raise a strong suspicion of malignancy, but the findings are not sufficient for a conclusive diagnosis. Specimens that are suspicious for a follicular or Hürthle cell neoplasm are excluded from this category (see Chaps. 5 and 6). For the category SFM, the morphologic changes are of such a degree that a malignancy is considered more likely than not. The target PPV of this category is 55–85%.[1]

Criteria

Suspicious for Papillary Carcinoma

Pattern A ("Patchy Nuclear Changes Pattern," Figs. 7.1 and 7.2)

The sample is moderately or highly cellular.

Benign follicular cells (arranged predominantly in macrofollicle fragments) are admixed with cells that have nuclear enlargement, nuclear pallor, nuclear grooves, nuclear membrane irregularity, and/or nuclear molding.

Intranuclear pseudoinclusions (INCIs) are rare or absent.

Pattern B ("Incomplete Nuclear Changes Pattern," Fig. 7.3)

The sample is sparsely, moderately, or highly cellular.

There is generalized mild-to-moderate nuclear enlargement with mild nuclear pallor.

Nuclear grooves are evident, but nuclear membrane irregularity and nuclear molding are minimal or absent.

Intranuclear pseudoinclusions are rare or absent.

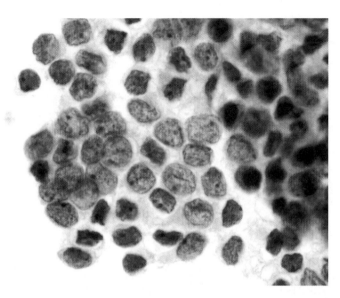

Figure 7.1. Suspicious for papillary thyroid carcinoma. This sheet of follicular cells displays some features of papillary carcinoma, including nuclear enlargement, powdery chromatin, nuclear membrane irregularity, nuclear grooves and molding, and small nucleoli. These changes were patchy, however, and other follicular cell sheets looked benign (ThinPrep, Papanicolaou stain).

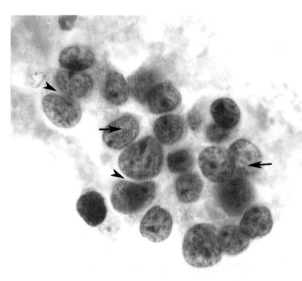

Figure 7.2. Suspicious for papillary thyroid carcinoma. This loose sheet of follicular cells demonstrates enlarged nuclei, powdery chromatin, nucleoli, and nuclear grooves. There are some questionable (i.e., small, poorly defined) intranuclear pseudoinclusions (*arrows*) and slight nuclear molding (*arrow heads*). These changes were patchy, however, and other follicular cells looked entirely benign (ThinPrep, Papanicolaou stain).

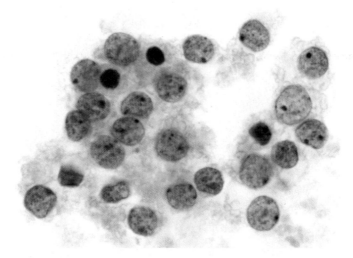

Figure 7.3. Suspicious for papillary thyroid carcinoma. In this specimen, there were generalized but mild nuclear changes. A loose sheet of follicular cells shows slightly enlarged nuclei, variable chromatin pallor, small but prominent nucleoli, nuclear grooves, and minimal molding (ThinPrep, Papanicolaou stain).

Pattern C ("Sparsely Cellular Specimen Pattern")

Many of the features of PTC (see Chap. 8) are present, but the sample is very sparsely cellular.

Pattern D ("Cystic Degeneration Pattern," Fig. 7.4)

There is evidence of cystic degeneration based on the presence of hemosiderin-laden macrophages.

Scattered groups and sheets of follicular cells have enlarged, pale nuclei and some have nuclear grooves, but INCIs are rare or absent.

There are occasional large, atypical, "histiocytoid" cells with enlarged nuclei and abundant vacuolated cytoplasm.

There are rare calcifications that resemble psammoma bodies.

Suspicious for Medullary Carcinoma (Figs. 7.5 and 7.6)

The sample is sparsely or moderately cellular.

There is a monomorphic population of noncohesive small or medium-sized cells with a high nuclear/cytoplasmic (N/C) ratio (? lymphoid lesion, ? medullary carcinoma).

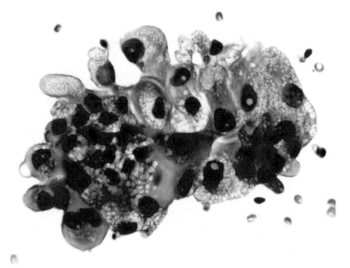

Figure 7.4. Suspicious for papillary thyroid carcinoma. There is a loose sheet of histiocytoid cells with vacuolated cytoplasm, occasional small nucleoli, and intranuclear pseudoinclusions (air-dried smear, Diff-Quik stain).

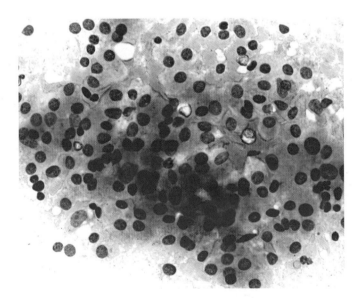

Figure 7.5. Suspicious for medullary thyroid carcinoma. There is a loose group of cells with relatively uniform nuclei; occasional larger nuclei with prominent nucleoli are present. The ill-defined cell borders make it difficult to discern the nature of the cytoplasm, the nuclear/cytoplasmic ratio, and the plasmacytoid contours of these cells. The stripped nuclei resemble small lymphocytes (air-dried smear, Diff-Quik stain).

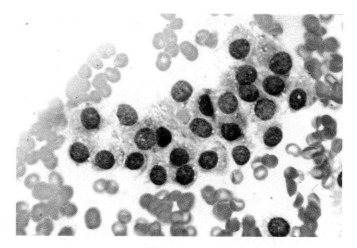

FIGURE 7.6. Suspicious for medullary thyroid carcinoma. This loose sheet of relatively uniform cells has vacuolated cytoplasm and ill-defined cell borders. The cells appear slightly degenerated, making it is difficult to discern their features with certainty (air-dried smear, Diff-Quik stain).

Nuclei are eccentrically located, with smudged chromatin due to suboptimal preservation; there are no discernible cytoplasmic granules.

There may be small fragments of amorphous material - colloid versus amyloid.

Suspicious for Lymphoma (Fig. 7.7)

The cellular sample is composed of numerous monomorphic small- to inter-mediate-sized lymphoid cells.

Or:

The sample is sparsely cellular and contains atypical lymphoid cells.

Suspicious for Malignancy, Not Otherwise Specified

(See Explanatory Notes.)

Explanatory Notes

Suspicious for Papillary Carcinoma

The criteria for the most common general patterns of "SFM, suspicious for PTC," are outlined above. In histologic sections, the diagnostic features of PTC can be patchy within a tumor nodule. This is reflected in the FNAs from those nodules. Unfortunately, this pattern is mimicked by a number of

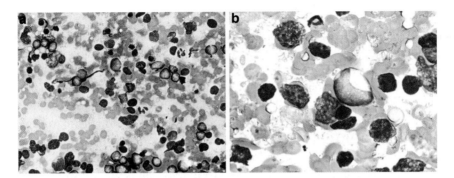

Figure 7.7. Suspicious for lymphoma. (**a**) This hemodilute sample is comprised exclusively of lymphoid cells, many of which appear poorly preserved. (**b**) At higher magnification, rare large atypical lymphoid cells are present, but most of the cells are disrupted and appear as bare nuclei. In the absence of immunophenotyping studies that demonstrate clonality, the findings are suspicious but not conclusive for malignant lymphoma (air-dried smear, Diff-Quik stain).

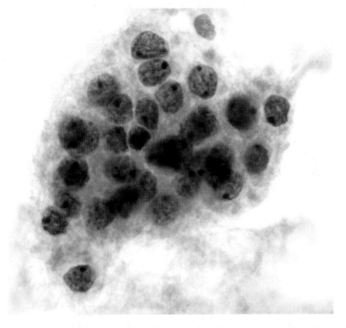

Figure 7.8. Suspicious for papillary thyroid carcinoma (patient with Hashimoto thyroiditis). There is a crowded group of follicular cells with nuclear enlargement, powdery chromatin, nuclear grooves and molding, and prominent nucleoli (ThinPrep, Papanicolaou stain).

benign conditions like LT, cystic degenerative changes, and radioiodine and carbimazole treatment. The nuclear changes of follicular cells in LT include focal enlargement, grooving, prominence of nucleoli, and chromatin clearing (Fig. 7.8). An abundance of lymphocytes and plasma cells does not exclude the possibility of a coexisting PTC.

Cyst lining cells associated with cystic degeneration have very characteristic features and can be diagnosed as benign in most cases.[8] These cells are typically elongated, with pale chromatin, and occasional intranuclear grooves, and relatively large nucleoli, and are virtually always associated with hemosiderin-laden macrophages and benign-appearing macrofollicle fragments. The spindle-shaped morphology of the cell and nucleus, reminiscent of reparative epithelium in cervical Pap specimens, is helpful in distinguishing these cells from PTC. In some cases, however, the cells are more difficult to distinguish from PTC.[8] A diagnosis of AUS is appropriate for some cases (see Chap. 4), but in their most marked form they can be highly worrisome, and an SFM interpretation may be warranted (Fig. 7.9).

In patients treated with radioactive iodine, carbimazole, or other pharmaceutical agents, nuclear atypia can be especially prominent.[9–11] In some patients, the nuclear changes can be extreme and raise the possibility of PTC or other malignancy.[10,11] As with cyst lining cells in their most extreme form, such cases warrant an SFM interpretation (Fig. 7.10).

Instead of being patchy, the nuclear changes are sometimes generalized but mild and incomplete. Again, such relatively subtle generalized changes are seen in some PTCs, particularly the follicular variant, but can be mimicked

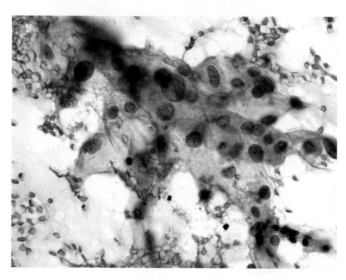

FIGURE 7.9. Suspicious for papillary thyroid carcinoma. Follicular cells adjacent to areas of infarction, hemorrhage, and cyst formation ("cyst lining cells") can have nuclear changes similar to those of papillary thyroid carcinoma. When nuclear enlargement, pallor, and grooves are widespread throughout the specimen, the diagnosis "suspicious for malignancy" may be unavoidable (smear, Papanicolaou stain).

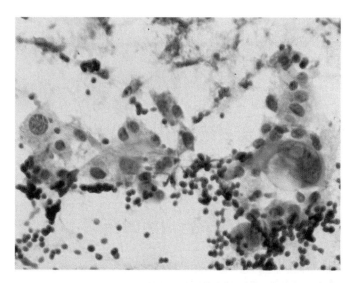

FIGURE 7.10. Suspicious for papillary thyroid carcinoma (patient treated with radioiodine for nodular goiter). These follicular cells demonstrate marked aniso-nucleosis, pale chromatin, and a prominent intranuclear cytoplasmic pseudoin-clusion. Although the findings may represent treatment effect, the possibility of papillary thyroid carcinoma cannot be excluded when the atypia is as marked as in this case (smear, Papanicolaou stain).

by benign lesions like a follicular adenoma. For this reason, when generalized but mild, the findings are best interpreted as SFM.

A number of histologic variants of PTC are distinguished by some sort of variation from the defining features of a classic PTC.[12–17] These include the follicular (Fig. 7.11), oncocytic (Figs. 7.12a and b), and columnar variants, as well as PTCs with cystic degeneration. Their morphologic differences are reflected in FNA specimens and can cause uncertainty in diagnosis. They may result in a sense of incompleteness or patchiness of expression of typical PTC features, and may be interpreted as SFM rather than malignant.

Hyalinizing trabecular tumor (HTT) shares many morphologic features with PTC, including nuclear grooves and abundant nuclear pseudoinclusions (Figs. 7.13a and b). Although it may be related to PTC,[18] it is generally dis-tinguished from PTC histologically based on its circumscription, trabecular growth pattern, and intratrabecular hyaline material.[19] These distinguishing features are difficult to appreciate by FNA, and many HTTs are interpreted as malignant or SFM.

Cystic PTCs, like other PTC variants, have unusual features that differ from those of the classic PTC, and their features can be obscured by blood and macrophages. Some contain large cells with abundant dense or vacuolated

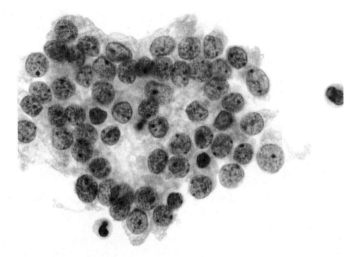

FIGURE 7.11. Suspicious for papillary thyroid carcinoma. This representative crowded group of follicular cells displays nuclear enlargement, variable chromatin pallor, rare nuclear grooves, small nucleoli, and focal molding (ThinPrep, Papanicolaou stain).

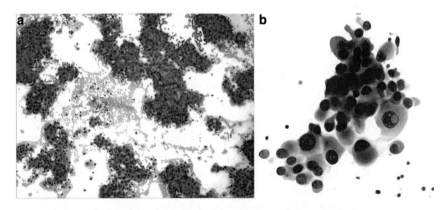

FIGURE 7.12. Suspicious for papillary thyroid carcinoma, oncocytic variant. (a) This low-magnification image reveals a hypercellular specimen with many groups of follicular that have abundant cytoplasm (air-dried smear, Diff-Quik stain). (b) High magnification confirms the presence of abundant cytoplasm and reveals intranuclear cytoplasmic pseudoinclusions (air-dried smear, Diff-Quik stain).

cytoplasm and pleomorphic nuclei ("histiocytoid cells") (Fig. 7.4). Such PTCs can be difficult to diagnose with certainty as malignant.[17,20]

Unfortunately, there are no reliable ancillary studies to distinguish PTC from its mimics in any given case.[21,22]

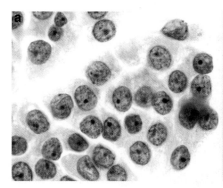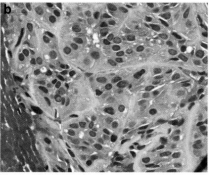

FIGURE 7.13. Suspicious for papillary thyroid carcinoma. (**a**) A loose sheet of follicular cells shows nuclear enlargement; pale, powdery chromatin; nuclear grooves; and prominent nucleoli (ThinPrep, Papanicolaou stain). (**b**) A cell block preparation from the FNA reveals the nested pattern of the atypical cells, along with their pale chromatin and obvious intranuclear cytoplasmic pseudoinclusions. The subsequent thyroidectomy revealed a hyalinizing trabecular tumor (cell block, H&E stain).

Suspicious for Medullary Carcinoma

Thyroid FNA has higher sensitivity for the detection of MTC than for PTC.[23] As with PTC, however, a specimen may be less than definitive for the diagnosis of MTC due to technical issues like cellularity and preservation (Fig. 7.6) or unusual cytomorphologic presentations.[24] In such cases, definitive diagnosis of MTC can be made if sufficient material is available for immunocytochemical stains (see Chap. 9), or if it is known that the patient has a markedly elevated serum calcitonin level.

Suspicious for Lymphoma

The inability to render a definitive diagnosis of diffuse large B-cell lymphoma is usually the result of technical limitations (e.g., suboptimal sampling and preservation, Fig. 7.7),[25] whereas a definitive diagnosis of a low-grade lymphoma (e.g., a MALT or low-grade follicular lymphoma) is intrinsically more challenging.[26–28] MALT lymphoma of the thyroid can be difficult to distinguish from LT without immunophenotyping by flow cytometry or immunocytochemistry, and a suspicious diagnosis may be prudent.[29] When a monomorphic population of small-to-intermediate sized cells predominates in a thyroid FNA, the suspicion of a low- or intermediate-grade lymphoma should be raised.

Flow cytometric demonstration of light chain restriction of B cells is often relied upon for a definitive diagnosis of lymphoma, but false-positive results have been reported in patients with LT.[30]

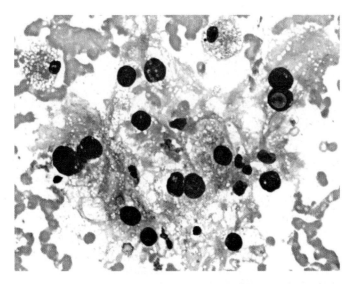

FIGURE 7.14. Suspicious for malignancy, cannot classify further. Scattered cells have abundant finely vacuolated cytoplasm, and one cell displays a large intra-nuclear cytoplasmic pseudoinclusion. The subsequent thyroidectomy showed metastatic renal cell carcinoma (air-dried smear, Diff-Quik stain).

Suspicious for Malignancy, Not Otherwise Specified

Other primary thyroid malignancies like undifferentiated (anaplastic) carcinoma and poorly differentiated carcinoma are encountered in the thyroid, as are metastases (Fig. 7.14). Although a diagnosis of malignancy is easily rendered in many cases, a specific diagnosis requires correlation with clinical and immunocytochemical findings. Suboptimal cellularity or preservation can lead to uncertainty and thus result in an SFM interpretation.

Management

The diagnosis "SFM, suspicious for papillary thyroid carcinoma" is an indication for surgery. The contribution of intraoperative frozen section and/or touch imprint after a "suspicious" FNA diagnosis is unclear. The accuracy of an intraoperative imprint of a thyroid lesion has not been investigated. When compared with intraoperative frozen section, FNA has been consistently shown to have at least a comparable, if not higher, sensitivity and PPV for PTC.[31,32] Consequently, some patients, in consultation with their surgeons, choose to undergo a total thyroidectomy, whereas others choose lobectomy with or without intraoperative frozen section. In the latter scenario, a completion thyroidectomy is done if the final histologic (or frozen section) diagnosis is PTC. A total thyroidectomy is considered for patients with large tumors (>4 cm) because of the increased risk of malignancy associated with tumors of that size.[21]

Ancillary serologic or immunohistochemical studies, which are of little value for patients with an FNA diagnosis of "suspicious for papillary thyroid carcinoma," can be very helpful for patients with the diagnosis "suspicious for MTC" or "suspicious for lymphoma." An elevated serum calcitonin level and/or a repeat FNA that shows strong immunoreactivity for chromogranin, synaptophysin, and calcitonin can convert an initial "suspicious for MTC" interpretation into a conclusively malignant interpretation. A repeat FNA to obtain cells for flow cytometric study is also likely to provide a definite diagnosis for patients with an initial "suspicious for lymphoma" interpretation.

Sample Reports

If an aspirate is interpreted as SFM, it is implied that the sample is adequate for evaluation. (An explicit statement of adequacy is optional.) Narrative comments that follow are used to specify which malignancy/ies the findings are suspicious for. A microscopic description is optional.

Example 1:
SUSPICIOUS FOR MALIGNANCY.
Suspicious for papillary thyroid carcinoma.

Example 2:
SUSPICIOUS FOR MALIGNANCY.
Suspicious for medullary thyroid carcinoma.
Note: Correlation with serum calcitonin level or re-aspiration for immunohistochemical studies might be helpful for definitive diagnosis if clinically indicated.

Example 3:
SUSPICIOUS FOR MALIGNANCY.
Suspicious for lymphoma.
Note: Re-aspiration for immunophenotyping studies by flow cytometry might be helpful for definitive diagnosis if clinically indicated.

References

1. Wang HH. Reporting thyroid fine-needle aspiration: Literature review and a proposal. *Diagn Cytopathol*. 2006;34(1):67-76.
2. Gharib H, Goellner JR, Johnson DA. Fine-needle aspiration cytology of the thyroid. A 12-year experience with 11, 000 biopsies. *Clin Lab Med*. 1993;13(3):699-709.

3. Renshaw AA. Accuracy of thyroid fine-needle aspiration using receiver operator characteristic curves. *Am J Clin Pathol.* 2001;116(4):477-482.
4. Tulecke MA, Wang HH. ThinPrep for cytologic evaluation of follicular thyroid lesions: correlation with histologic findings. *Diagn Cytopathol.* 2004;30(1):7-13.
5. Yassa L, Cibas ES, Benson CB, et al. Long-term assessment of a multidisciplinary approach to thyroid nodule diagnostic evaluation. *Cancer.* 2007;111(6):508-516.
6. Zhang Y, Fraser JL, Wang HH. Morphologic predictors of papillary carcinoma on fine-needle aspiration of thyroid with ThinPrep preparations. *Diagn Cytopathol.* 2001;24(6): 378-383.
7. Weber D, Brainard J, Chen L. Atypical epithelial cells, cannot exclude papillary carcinoma, in fine needle aspiration of the thyroid. *Acta Cytol.* 2008;52(3):320-324.
8. Faquin WC, Cibas ES, Renshaw AA. "Atypical" cells in fine-needle aspiration biopsy specimens of benign thyroid cysts. *Cancer.* 2005;105(2):71-79.
9. Smejkal V, Smejkalova E, Rosa M, Zeman V, Smetana K. Cytologic changes simulating malignancy in thyrotoxic goiters treated with carbimazole. *Acta Cytol.* 1985;29:173-178.
10. Granter SR, Cibas ES. Cytologic findings in thyroid nodules after 131iodine treatment of hyperthyroidism. *Am J Clin Pathol.* 1997;107:20-25.
11. Centeno BA, Szyfelbein WM, Daniels GH, Vickery AL. Fine-needle aspiration biopsy of the thyroid gland in patients with prior Graves' disease treated with radioactive iodine: morphologic findings and potential pitfalls. *Acta Cytol.* 1996;40:1189-1197.
12. Liu J, Singh B, Tallini G, et al. Follicular variant of papillary thyroid carcinoma: a clinicopathologic study of a problematic entity. *Cancer.* 2006;107(6):1255-1264.
13. Das DK, Mallik MK, Sharma P, et al. Papillary thyroid carcinoma and its variants in fine needle aspiration smears A cytomorphologic study with special reference to tall cell variant. *Acta Cytol.* 2004;48(3):325-336.
14. Gupta S, Sodhani P, Jain S, Kumar N. Morphologic spectrum of papillary carcinoma of the thyroid: role of cytology in identifying the variants. *Acta Cytol.* 2004;48(6):795-800.
15. Ylagan LR, Dehner LP, Huettner PC, Lu D. Columnar cell variant of papillary thyroid carcinoma Report of a case with cytologic findings. *Acta Cytol.* 2004;48(1):73-77.
16. Goellner JR, Johnson DA. Cytology of cystic papillary carcinoma of the thyroid. *Acta Cytol.* 1982;26(6):797-808.
17. Renshaw AA. "Histiocytoid" cells in fine-needle aspirations of papillary carcinoma of the thyroid: frequency and significance of an under-recognized cytologic pattern. *Cancer.* 2002;96(4):240-243.
18. Papotti M, Volante M, Giuliano A, et al. RET/PTC activation in hyalinizing trabecular tumors of the thyroid. *Am J Surg Pathol.* 2000;24(12):1615-1621.
19. DeLellis RA, Lloyd RV, Heitz PU, Eng C, eds. *World Health Organization classification of tumours. Pathology and genetics of tumours of endocrine organs.* Lyon: IARC Press; 2004.
20. Castro-Gomez L, Cordova-Ramirez S, Duarte-Torres R, Alonso de Ruiz P, Hurtado-Lopez LM. Cytologic criteria of cystic papillary carcinoma of the thyroid. *Acta Cytol.* 2003;47(4):590-594.
21. Cooper DS, Doherty GM, Haugen BR, et al. Management guidelines for patients with thyroid nodules and differentiated thyroid cancer. *Thyroid.* 2006;16(2):109-142.
22. Filie AC, Asa SL, Geisinger KR, et al. Utilization of ancillary studies in thyroid fine needle aspirates: a synopsis of the National Cancer Institute Thyroid Fine Needle Aspiration State of the Science Conference. *Diagn Cytopathol.* 2008;36(6):438-441.
23. Giard RW, Hermans J. Use and accuracy of fine-needle aspiration cytology in histologically proven thyroid carcinoma: an audit using a national nathology database. *Cancer.* 2000;90(6):330-334.

24. Papaparaskeva K, Nagel H, Droese M. Cytologic diagnosis of medullary carcinoma of the thyroid gland. *Diagn Cytopathol.* 2000;22(6):351-358.
25. Zeppa P, Marino G, Troncone G, et al. Fine-needle cytology and flow cytometry immunophenotyping and subclassification of non-Hodgkin lymphoma: a critical review of 307 cases with technical suggestions. *Cancer.* 2004;102(1):55-65.
26. Chhieng DC, Cohen JM, Cangiarella JF. Cytology and immunophenotyping of low- and intermediate-grade B-cell non-Hodgkin's lymphomas with a predominant small-cell component: a study of 56 cases. *Diagn Cytopathol.* 2001;24(2):90-97.
27. Crapanzano JP, Lin O. Cytologic findings of marginal zone lymphoma. *Cancer.* 2003;99(5):301-309.
28. Matsushima AY, Hamele-Bena D, Osborne BM. Fine-needle aspiration biopsy findings in marginal zone B cell lymphoma. *Diagn Cytopathol.* 1999;20(4):190-198.
29. Lerma E, Arguelles R, Rigla M, et al. Comparative findings of lymphocytic thyroiditis and thyroid lymphoma. *Acta Cytol.* 2003;47(4):575-580.
30. Chen HI, Akpolat I, Mody DR, et al. Restricted kappa/lambda light chain ratio by flow cytometry in germinal center B cells in Hashimoto thyroiditis. *Am J Clin Pathol.* 2006;125(1):42-48.
31. Hamburger JI, Husain M. Contribution of intraoperative pathology evaluation to surgical management of thyroid nodules. *Endocrinol Metab Clin North Am.* 1990;19(3):509-522.
32. Lee TI, Yang HJ, Lin SY, et al. The accuracy of fine-needle aspiration biopsy and frozen section in patients with thyroid cancer. *Thyroid.* 2002;12(7):619-626.

Chapter 8

Papillary Thyroid Carcinoma and Variants

Manon Auger, Edward B. Stelow, Grace C.H. Yang,
Miguel A. Sanchez, Sylvia L. Asa, and Virginia A. Livolsi

Background

Papillary thyroid carcinoma (PTC) is the most common malignant neoplasm of the thyroid, accounting for approximately 80% of all cancers at this site. It occurs in all age groups, including children, with a peak incidence in the third to fourth decades, and the M:F ratio is 1:3. Risk factors include external radiation to the neck during childhood, ionizing radiation, genetic factors, and nodular hyperplasia. PTC usually presents as a thyroid nodule, often discovered incidentally on routine examination; rarely, patients present with metastatic disease in the neck lymph nodes. PTC spreads via lymphatics to the regional lymph nodes and, less frequently, to the lungs. It generally carries a good prognosis; death secondary to PTC is rare.[1]

A malignant thyroid FNA diagnosis accounts for 4–8% of all thyroid FNAs,[2-4] the majority of them PTCs. When a definite diagnosis of PTC is made by FNA, 96–100% prove to be PTC on histologic follow-up.[2,3,5-7] Conventional PTCs are characterized histologically by numerous papillae lined by cuboidal to low columnar follicular cells with characteristic nuclear features (see below). Although traditionally considered the most common type of PTC, conventional PTC is diminishing in relative frequency as compared to PTC variants, especially in view of the increasing awareness and recognition of the follicular variant of PTC (FVPTC).

Syed Z. Ali and Edmund S. Cibas (eds.), *The Bethesda System for Reporting Thyroid Cytopathology*, DOI 10.1007/ 978-0-387-87666-5_8,

Papillary Thyroid Carcinoma (Figs. 8.1–8.13)

Definition

PTC is a malignant epithelial tumor derived from thyroid follicular epithelium and displays characteristic nuclear alterations. Papillary architecture may be present but is not required for the diagnosis.

Criteria (for All Types of PTC, Conventional and Variants)

Follicular cells are arranged in papillae and/or syncytial-like monolayers.
   Swirling sheets ("onion-skin" or "cartwheel" patterns) are sometimes seen.
   The altered follicular cells exhibit characteristic nuclear features:
      Enlarged nuclei
      Oval or irregularly shaped, sometimes molded nuclei
      Longitudinal nuclear grooves
      Intranuclear cytoplasmic pseudoinclusions (INCI)
      Pale nuclei with powdery chromatin ("Orphan Annie" nuclei)
      Marginally placed micronucleoli, solitary or multiple
   Psammoma bodies are sometimes present.
   Multinucleated giant cells are common.

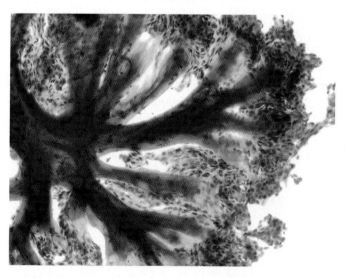

FIGURE 8.1. Papillary thyroid carcinoma. True papillary tissue fragments, comprised of fibrovascular cores lined by neoplastic cells, are seen in the conventional type of papillary thyroid carcinoma (smear, Papanicolaou stain).

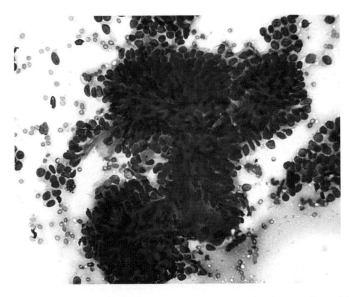

FIGURE 8.2. Papillary thyroid carcinoma. There is marked crowding of the neoplastic cells that line the papillae (smear, Diff-Quik stain).

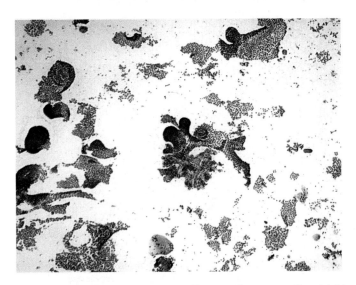

FIGURE 8.3. Papillary thyroid carcinoma. Preparations are often highly cellular and composed of numerous monolayer sheets and occasional papillary-like fragments (smear, Papanicolaou stain).

The amount of colloid is variable and may be stringy, ropy, or "bubble-gum"-like.

Hürthle cell (oncocytic) metaplasia is sometimes seen.

Squamous metaplasia is sometimes seen.

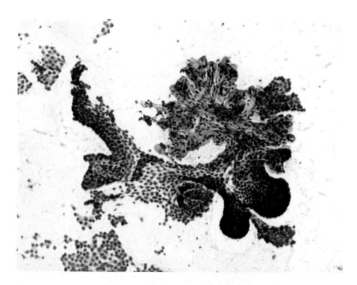

FIGURE 8.4. Papillary thyroid carcinoma. There is a mix of flat sheets and rounded, papillary-like fragments without fibrovascular cores (smear, Papanicolaou stain).

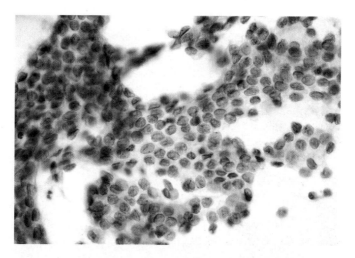

FIGURE 8.5. Papillary thyroid carcinoma. Monolayer sheets with a syncytial-like appearance are characteristic of papillary thyroid carcinoma. These flat sheets resemble those of benign follicular nodules; attention to the nuclear features is essential for this distinction (smear, Papanicolaou stain).

Explanatory Notes

Although certain typical nuclear alterations help define PTC, none of them are diagnostic of PTC in isolation or low frequency. Only when relatively widespread and in combination are they diagnostic of PTC in an FNA.[8,9]

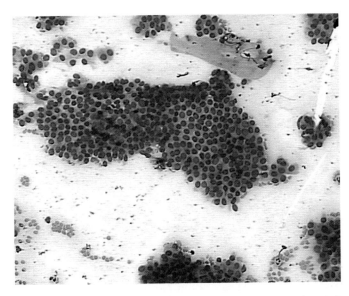

FIGURE 8.6. Papillary thyroid carcinoma. Monolayer sheets of neoplastic cells are associated with thick, sticky colloid (smear, Diff-Quik stain).

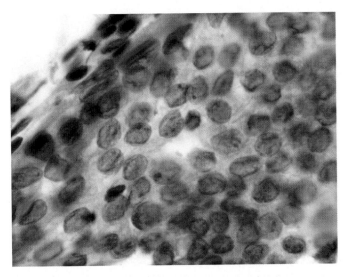

FIGURE 8.7. Papillary thyroid carcinoma. Close inspection at high magnification shows frequent nuclear grooves, finely textured (powdery) chromatin, and micronucleoli (smear, Papanicolaou stain).

The minimum criteria and number of altered cells necessary for an unequivocal diagnosis is uncertain and probably not definable, either cytologically or histopathologically, because of the variation in diagnostic thresholds among observers.[10–15] If, in the judgment of the cytologist, a case has some features

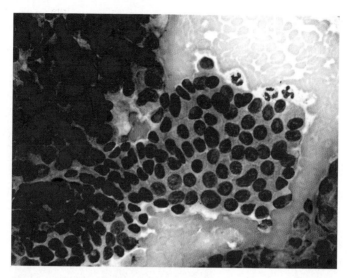

Figure 8.8. Papillary thyroid carcinoma. Nuclear grooves are less conspicuous with air-dried preparations as compared with alcohol-fixed slides (smear, Diff-Quik stain).

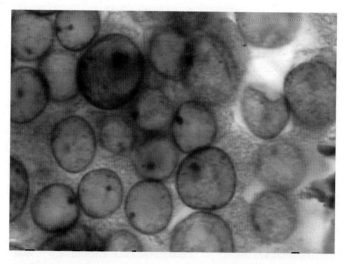

Figure 8.9. Papillary thyroid carcinoma. "Orphan Annie eyed" nuclei are very pale, with powdery chromatin and micronucleoli (smear, Papanicolaou stain).

of PTC but falls short of an unequivocal diagnosis, it is interpreted as "Suspicious for PTC" or "Atypia of undetermined significance (AUS)" (see Chaps. 7 and 4 respectively), depending on the quality and quantity of the changes and the reviewer's resulting level of suspicion for PTC.

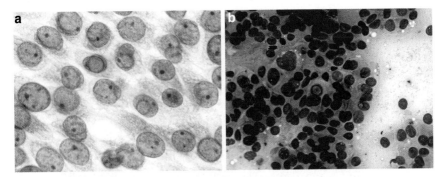

FIGURE 8.10. Papillary thyroid carcinoma. (a) Intranuclear cytoplasmic pseudoinclusions (INCIs) and micronucleoli are shown. Note that the two INCIs share the same aqua color and granular texture as the surrounding cytoplasm (smear, Papanicolaou stain). (b) A large INCI occupying most of the nucleus is seen in the center. The remaining nuclei show variation in size and shape (smear, Diff-Quik stain).

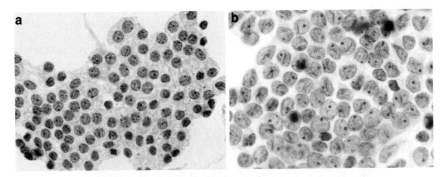

FIGURE 8.11. Comparison of benign follicular cells with the cells of papillary thyroid carcinoma. (a) Benign follicular cells (nodular goiter). (b) Compared with those of the benign follicular cells, the nuclei of papillary carcinoma are larger, paler, more crowded, and more irregular in contour. (a and b, ThinPrep, Papanicolaou stain).

On FNA preparations, the cells of a PTC are typically arranged in syncytial-like flat sheets ("monolayers") with crowded and overlapping nuclei. The crowding and overlapping of PTC nuclei is often impressive, with conspicuous molding of the nuclei. Crowding, overlapping, and molding are important diagnostic features that help distinguish them from benign follicular cells. The architectural pattern varies depending on the type of PTC (see below), and includes a variety of patterns: true papillary fragments (those having a fibrovascular core), papillary-like fragments (papillary shape but lacking a fibrovascular core), microfollicles, swirls (sometimes called an "onion-skin" or "cartwheel" pattern), as well as the monolayered sheet previously mentioned. A pattern of predominantly isolated cells is highly unusual. The monolayered sheet is characteristic of

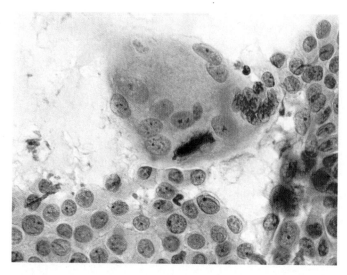

FIGURE 8.12. Papillary thyroid carcinoma. A multinucleated giant cell is seen adjacent to a monolayer of tumor cells. Although multinucleated giant cells are often seen in PTCs, they are non-specific (smear, Papanicolaou stain).

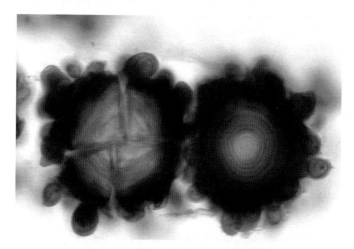

FIGURE 8.13. Papillary thyroid carcinoma. Psammoma bodies have concentric rings and are lined by atypical cells with oval, pale nuclei (smear, Papanicolaou stain).

PTC but mimics the flat sheet of a macrofollicle fragment typical of benign follicular nodules, such as those commonly seen in nodular hyperplasia. The distinction necessitates particular attention to the arrangement of the cells in the sheets (evenly spaced vs. crowded) and their nuclear features to avoid a false-negative diagnosis.

The cells of PTC vary in size, from medium to large, and shape (cuboidal, columnar, polygonal, sometimes spindle-shaped, and rarely "histiocytoid")[16].

Cell borders are usually well-demarcated. The amount and texture of cytoplasm also vary greatly. In some cases, the cells have scant cytoplasm, but abundant oncocytic (granular) cytoplasm is common as a focal finding. When extensive, it signals an oncocytic variant of PTC. Changes resembling squamous metaplasia (moderate to abundant dense cytoplasm and cells that fit together like paving stones) are also seen as a focal finding in PTC. Hyperkeratinized squamous cells (orangeophilic cytoplasm with the Papanicolaou stain) and keratin pearls, however, are rare.

The defining features of PTC are seen in the nuclei. PTC nuclei can be round or oval, but they are often highly irregular in contour; the irregularity of nuclear contours is often one of the first clues to the diagnosis. The chromatin of a PTC nucleus is usually pale and powdery rather than dark and coarsely textured like a benign follicular cell nucleus. The pallor is the greatest in formalin-fixed tissue, which renders the nucleus practically empty in appearance, like the empty eyes of the cartoon character Orphan Annie. INCIs are seen in 50–100% of aspirates of PTC. They are not specific for PTC because they are seen in medullary thyroid carcinoma, poorly differentiated carcinoma, anaplastic thyroid carcinoma, and, very rarely, benign thyroid nodules (e.g., nodular goiter, follicular adenoma, and lymphocytic thyroiditis). INCI should therefore always be interpreted in light of the other architectural and nuclear features in the case. Ultrastructurally, INCI are membrane-bound spheroidal masses of cytoplasm that protrude into the nuclei. Thus, a true INCI displays the same color/texture of cytoplasm and is sharply bordered by a rim of condensed chromatin. These features help to distinguish INCI from its common mimics: degenerative and artifactual vacuoles, fixation artifacts, and superimposed red blood cells.

Nuclear grooves are another hallmark of PTC.[17] They are best seen with alcohol-fixed, Papanicolaou-stained preparations and are less conspicuous with air-dried, Romanowsky-stained smears. Nuclear grooves and INCI are manifestations of the increased deformability of the PTC nucleus; a nuclear groove, for example, results from a nucleus folded onto itself.[18] Although characteristic of PTC, nuclear grooves are not specific and can be seen in a variety of other thyroid neoplasms and non-neoplastic conditions. For this reason, they should not be relied upon in isolation to make a diagnosis of PTC.

Multinucleated giant cells are commonly seen in aspirates of PTC, even when cystic degeneration is not present. Although common, they are not specific for PTC, and similar cells are seen in other conditions, benign and malignant. The cells can be very large, and their nuclei can vary in number from few to many. They are not malignant, but rather a response of the host immune system to the malignancy. Psammoma bodies (PBs) are seen less frequently in FNA samples of PTC (4–20% of cases) than in histologic specimens (40–60%). They can be solitary or multiple, isolated or attached to cells. PBs alone (i.e., not associated with altered cells) are non-specific and can be seen in medullary thyroid carcinoma, lymphocytic thyroiditis, Graves' disease, and even nodular goiter. Calcifications resembling PBs occur in benign Hürthle cell nodules and adenomas and represent calcification of colloid. The positive predictive value (PPV) for PTC of PBs in isolation is 50%; when seen in association with the cytologic features of PTC, the PPV is 100%.[19]

The background usually contains relatively scant colloid, but some variants (see below) can have abundant colloid. Colloid may be watery or dense and stringy with ropy strands ("bubble-gum" colloid). The background is usually clean; necrotic debris is extremely uncommon. Hemosiderin-laden macrophages, representing hemorrhage and cystic change, are common in PTC and can be prominent. Variable numbers of lymphocytes can be seen due to an underlying lymphocytic thyroiditis. When lymphocytes predominate, a Warthin-like variant of PTC should be considered (see below). Caution should be exercised when nuclear abnormalities are seen in follicular cell clusters with intimately admixed lymphocytes, as these nuclear changes may be reactive and not malignant.

Given an adequate sample, it is relatively straightforward to diagnose PTC by FNA. Although false-negative and false-positive diagnoses occasionally occur, they can be minimized by adopting a conservative approach to a sparsely cellular or otherwise suboptimal specimen. This recommendation applies as well to cases with focal or limited nuclear changes.

Variants of Papillary Thyroid Carcinoma

A significant proportion of PTCs exhibit variant architectural and/or cytologic features from those of the conventional PTC (Figs. 8.14–8.26). Variants of PTC, by definition, have the essential nuclear features of PTC but a different architectural pattern, unusual cytoplasmic features, or different background features, such as the quantity and texture of the colloid and the presence or absence of a prominent lymphoplasmacytic infiltrate.

Some of the PTC variants have a different clinical prognosis than the conventional PTC, but distinction at the time of FNA is not necessary because the initial treatment (usually total thyroidectomy) is the same. Precise subtyping may not be possible because the predominant pattern may not have been sampled in the FNA (as many PTCs show more than one growth pattern) and because some of these variants are very rare and familiarity with their morphologic features may be unrealistic. Nonetheless, the architectural and cytologic features that distinguish these lesions from conventional PTC histologically are often observed cytologically. If for no other reason, awareness of the phenotypic characteristics of the various subtypes can diminish the risk of misdiagnosing them.

Follicular Variant (Figs. 8.14–8.16)

Definition

The follicular variant of PTC (FVPTC) is a PTC in which the tumor is completely or almost completely composed of small to medium-sized follicles lined by cells with the nuclear features of a PTC.

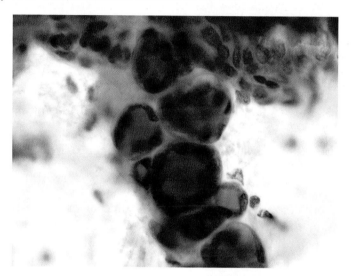

FIGURE 8.14. Papillary thyroid carcinoma, follicular variant. The neoplastic cells are arranged mostly as microfollicles (smear, Papanicolaou stain).

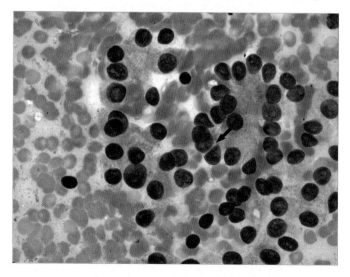

FIGURE 8.15. Papillary thyroid carcinoma, follicular variant. The cells are arranged mostly as microfollicles. Note the molding of adjacent nuclei (*arrow*) and the irregular spacing of the neoplastic cells (smear, Diff-Quik stain).

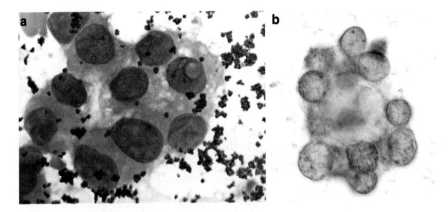

Figure 8.16. Papillary thyroid carcinoma, follicular variant. (**a**) The characteristic nuclear features of PTC are seen (e.g., nuclear enlargement and intranuclear pseudoinclusions.) (smear, Diff-Quik stain). (**b**) A microfollicle is composed of several enlarged, crowded, oval, and pale nuclei (smear; Papanicolaou stain).

Background

It has long been recognized that some PTCs are composed primarily if not exclusively of follicles rather than papillae.[20,21] FVPTC is now the most common variant of PTC and represents nearly 30% of PTCs in some series. It behaves clinically in a manner indistinguishable from conventional PTC. The vast majority of these tumors are composed of microfollicles; however, some FVPTCs are composed of normal-sized follicles. Tumors composed predominantly of macrofollicles are considered a different and distinct subset of PTC (see below). The degree to which the nuclear features are displayed in a FVPTC varies from case to case. Some FVPTCs have prominent classic nuclear features of PTC, but in others the features are only partially and focally displayed. For this reason, a distinction among the various "follicular-patterned" lesions of the thyroid (e.g., nodular goiter, follicular adenoma, FVPTC) is often troublesome.[14]

Criteria

Samples are usually hypercellular, with syncytial-like fragments containing microfollicles ("rosettes"). Dispersed microfollicular clusters, isolated neoplastic follicles, and some sheets with branched irregular contours may also be present.

Some colloid may be present, typically dense-staining, thick, and sometimes within neoplastic follicles.

In contrast to conventional PTC, the nuclear changes are often subtle.

The following features are usually absent or inconspicuous: papillary and papillary-like fragments, multinucleated giant cells, INCIs, psammoma bodies, marked cystic change.

Explanatory Notes

FVPTC typically show cells with nuclear enlargement and chromatin clearing, but nuclear grooves and INCIs are less common than in conventional PTC, and many FVPTCs are interpreted as "suspicious for papillary carcinoma" rather than unequivocally malignant.[22-25] For the same reasons, FVPTC can be difficult to distinguish from the other cellular follicular aspirates, and many are diagnosed as "follicular neoplasm/suspicious for follicular neoplasm." Particular attention must be paid to the presence of ovoid, pear-shaped, and cerebriform (or raisin-shaped) nuclei. Prudence is recommended, however, and current practice suggests that only the cases with definitive nuclear features of PTC should be diagnosed unequivocally on FNA.

Macrofollicular Variant (Figs. 8.17, 8.18)

Definition

The macrofollicular variant is a PTC in which over 50% of the follicles are arranged as macrofollicles.[1]

Criteria

The sample consists of monolayered (two-dimensional) sheets of atypical epithelium and/or variably sized follicles.

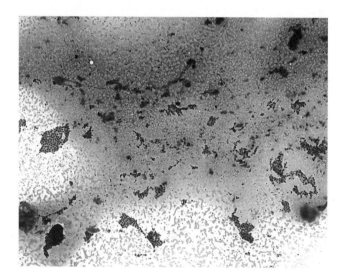

FIGURE 8.17. Papillary thyroid carcinoma, macrofollicular variant. The neoplastic cells resemble those of a benign thyroid nodule at scanning magnification. In such cases there can be abundant thin colloid and relatively few sheets of cells. The difference lies in the nuclear features, which are better appreciated at high magnification (smear, Diff-Quik stain).

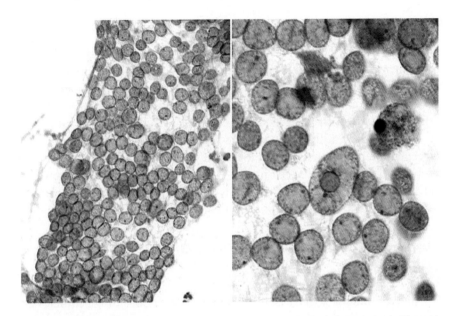

Figure 8.18. Papillary thyroid carcinoma, macrofollicular variant. *Left,* There is a large sheet of tumor cells with crowded, "Orphan Annie eye" nuclei; *Right,* An intranuclear pseudoinclusion is present in the large oval nucleus. Note also the peripheral micronucleoli (smear, Papanicolaou stain).

Convincing nuclear changes of PTC must be present for a definite interpretation of malignancy.

In contrast to conventional PTC, the diagnostic nuclear features are often more subtle (as with FVPTC).

Abundant thin colloid or fragments of thick colloid may also be present.

Explanatory Notes

The differential diagnosis of a macrofollicular variant of PTC includes the benign follicular nodule seen with nodular goiter and the follicular adenoma of macrofollicular type.[25,26] The macrofollicular variant is easily overlooked at low magnification due to the abundance of thin colloid, the low cellularity, and the subtle and focal nuclear atypia.[26] Thus, careful attention to nuclear features is necessary for all benign-appearing thyroid aspirates.

Cystic Variant (Figs. 8.19, 8.20)

Definition

The cystic variant is a PTC that is predominantly cystic, comprised of thin, watery fluid, abundant histiocytes, and hypervacuolated tumor cells.

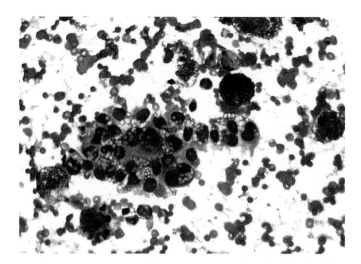

FIGURE 8.19. Papillary thyroid carcinoma, cystic variant. There is prominent cystic change with numerous hemosiderin-laden macrophages. Monolayered sheets of neoplastic cells show nuclear features of PTC (smear, Diff-Quik stain).

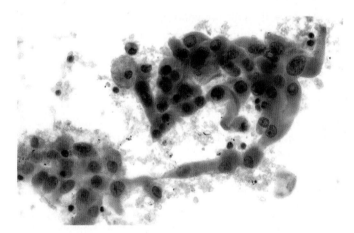

FIGURE 8.20. Papillary thyroid carcinoma, cystic variant. Cystic changes with macrophages are apparent. The neoplastic cells have more abundant granular cytoplasm than usual, a non-specific finding in this case. Diagnostic nuclear features of papillary thyroid carcinoma are recognizable, including nuclear enlargement and overlap and occasional intranuclear pseudoinclusions (smear, Papanicolaou stain).

Criteria

The neoplastic cells are typically arranged in small groups with irregular borders; sheets, papillae, or follicles may also be present.

Tumor cells look "histiocytoid" (hypervacuolated).

Macrophages, often containing hemosiderin, are present.

There is a variable amount of thin or watery colloid.

Convincing nuclear changes of PTC must be present for a definite diagnosis of malignancy.

In contrast to conventional PTC, the fine powdery chromatin is usually less prominent, presumably due to cellular degeneration, and cellular swirls/onion-skin appearance and cart-wheel arrangement of the follicular cells are more frequently seen.

Explanatory Notes

PTC is the most common malignant neoplasm of the thyroid to undergo cystic change. The amount of cystic change can vary, and approximately 10% of PTCs are almost entirely cystic.[21] Histologically, most cystic PTCs retain a papillary architecture.

FNAs of cystic PTC show varying proportions of macrophages, colloid, and neoplastic cells.[27] The neoplastic cells have more abundant, granular or vacuolated cytoplasm than the conventional PTC. The tumor cells frequently appear more rigid and polygonal than normal follicular cells and display enlarged, oval to irregularly-shaped nuclei with prominent nuclear grooves and INCIs. The more subtle nuclear features of PTC, like "powdery" chromatin or clearing, are often less apparent. Whereas some aspirates have abundant neoplastic cells and are readily interpreted as PTC, others have no neoplastic cells at all and are best interpreted as "Nondiagnostic; cyst fluid only." Indeed, cystic PTC has long been recognized as a possible cause for false-negative thyroid FNAs.

It should also be noted that atypical cells with some of the features of PTC are sometimes seen in benign follicular nodules with cystic change.[28] These cells are frequently arranged in streaming sheets. They have enlarged nuclei, nucleoli, nuclear pallor, and occasional nuclear grooves. Their benign nature is betrayed by their elongated shape and the lack of nuclear crowding and INCIs. In some cases, however, the nuclear changes can be extreme. Not surprisingly, some cases are best diagnosed as "suspicious for papillary carcinoma" or AUS/FLUS (see Chaps. 7 and 4, respectively).

Oncocytic Variant (Figs. 8.21, 8.22)

Definition

The oncocytic variant is a thyroid tumor with the nuclear changes characteristic of PTC but composed predominantly of oncocytic cells (polygonal cells with abundant granular cytoplasm).

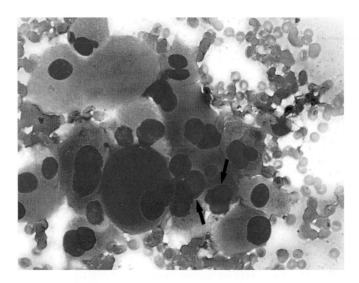

Figure 8.21. Papillary thyroid carcinoma, oncocytic variant. The neoplasm is composed throughout of oncocytic (Hürthle-like) cells that have abundant granular cytoplasm. Several intranuclear pseudoinclusions are visible (*arrows*) (smears, Diff-Quik stain).

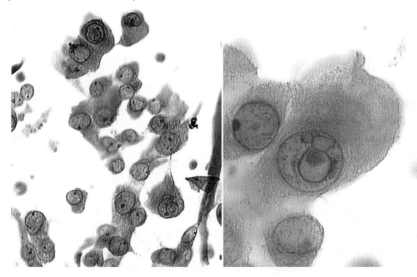

Figure 8.22. Papillary thyroid carcinoma, oncocytic variant. *Left*, Loosely cohesive polygonal oncocytic (Hürthle-like) cells have atypical clear nuclei with eccentric micronucleoli and rare intranuclear pseudoinclusions. *Right*, Multiple small and large intranuclear pseudoinclusions can be seen in a large oncocytic cell with abundant granular cytoplasm (smears, Papanicolaou stain).

Criteria

The sample is composed predominantly of oncocytic cells, arranged in papillae, sheets, or as isolated cells.

Convincing diagnostic nuclear changes of PTC must be present for a definite diagnosis of PTC.

Lymphocytes are absent or few in number.

Explanatory Notes

Focal oncocytic (also called Hürthle cell or oxyphilic cell) change is seen in many PTCs, including the conventional PTC. Only when the changes are widespread does the tumor merit distinction as an oncocytic variant of PTC.[29,30] Aspirates of the oncocytic variant of PTC resemble those from Hürthle cell proliferations, including Hürthle cell neoplasms. The characteristic nuclear features of PTC, therefore, must be searched for whenever an aspirate is composed predominantly of Hürthle cells (oncocytes). Non-PTC Hürthle cell (oncocytic) lesions generally have rounder nuclei and more prominent nucleoli than the oncocytic variant of PTC. In addition, non-PTC Hürthle cell (oncocytic) proliferations may have nuclear grooves and slight nuclear pallor, but INCIs are very rarely seen. Lymphocytes are typically absent in FNAs of the oncocytic variant of PTC; if present in large numbers, a Warthin-like variant of PTC should be considered.

Warthin-like Variant

Definition

The Warthin-like variant of PTC is a circumscribed thyroid tumor with papillary architecture and lymphoid follicles that mimics a Warthin tumor of the parotid gland. The neoplastic cells have abundant granular cytoplasm and the nuclear features of PTC.

Criteria

The neoplastic cells are oncocytic and arranged in papillae and as dispersed cells.

A lymphoplasmacytic background is present. The lymphocytes permeate the fibrovascular stalk and are intimately associated with the tumor cells.

Convincing nuclear changes of PTC must be present for a definite diagnosis of malignancy.

Explanatory Notes

Because of the mixture of oncocytes and lymphocytes, FNAs from the Warthin-like variant of PTC resemble those from Hashimoto thyroiditis.[31] The Hürthle (oncocytic) cells of Hashimoto thyroiditis, however, typically have round nuclei with a prominent single nucleolus; the nuclei of PTC (including the Warthin-like variant), by contrast, are more irregular in contour and nucleoli are less prominent. The Hürthle cells in Hashimoto thyroiditis may show nuclear clearing and grooves, but papillary fragments and INCIs are usually not seen.

Tall Cell Variant (Figs. 8.23, 8.24)

Definition

The tall cell variant (TCV) is an aggressive form of PTC composed of papillae lined by a single layer of elongated ("tall") tumor cells (their height is at least three times their width) with abundant dense granular cytoplasm and the typical nuclear changes of PTC. Tall cells with abundant cytoplasm should account for at least 50% of the tumor for it to be classified as a TCV.[32]

Criteria

The neoplastic cells have an elongated shape, with a height-to-width ratio of at least 3:1.

The neoplastic cells have distinct cell borders and are arranged in papillary fragments.

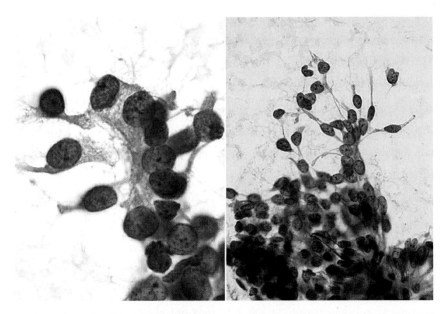

FIGURE 8.23. Papillary thyroid carcinoma, tall cell variant of PTC. *Left*, Tall cells with oval, clear nuclei and elongated cytoplasm. *Right*, Tall cells are often found at the edge of tumor fragments (smears, Papanicolaou stain).

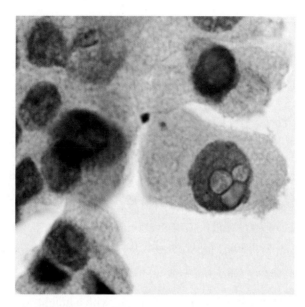

Figure 8.24. Papillary thyroid carcinoma, tall cell variant. "Soap bubble-like" intranuclear pseudoinclusions are often seen in the tall cell variant of papillary thyroid carcinoma (ThinPrep, Papanicolaou stain).

Some lymphocytes may be present.

Convincing nuclear changes of PTC must be present for a definite diagnosis of malignancy.

In contrast to conventional PTC:
- the nuclear chromatin is sometimes less powdery and more granular
- psammoma bodies are fewer in number
- INCI tend to be more frequent and more often multiple within one nucleus, imparting a "soap bubble" appearance to the nucleus

Explanatory Notes

The TCV tends to occur in elderly patients and is more frequent in men, than are the other PTCs. It is often presented as a large and bulky tumor, often with an extrathyroidal extension and vascular invasion. It is more aggressive than the conventional PTC and has a higher incidence of local recurrence and distant metastasis.[1]

The TCV is easily recognized as PTC due to the abundance of papillary fragments and the prominent INCIs.[33] It is not always possible to subtype the tumor as a TCV, however, because the neoplastic cells are often cohesive, making assessment of the individual cell features difficult.

Columnar Cell Variant (Figs. 8.25, 8.26)

Definition

The columnar cell variant is a rare aggressive variant of PTC, characterized by columnar cells with hyperchromatic, oval, and stratified nuclei and supranuclear or subnuclear cytoplasmic vacuoles. The cells are typically arranged in papillae, but trabeculae and follicles can also be seen.

Criteria

Smears are cellular and generally lack colloid.

The neoplastic cells are arranged as papillae, clusters, and flat sheets, sometimes with small tubular structures.

The nuclei are elongated and stratified.[34]

Convincing nuclear changes of PTC must be present for a definitive diagnosis of malignancy.

In contrast to conventional PTC:

- the nuclear features of PTC (grooves, INCI) are focal and less prominent
- the nuclear chromatin tends to be hyperchromatic rather than pale and powdery
- colloid and cystic change (macrophages) are typically not seen

Explanatory Notes

Because the nuclei of the columnar cell variant are darker than those of the typical PTC, and because the other typical nuclear features of PTC are less frequent, the neoplastic cells of the columnar cell variant may be mistaken

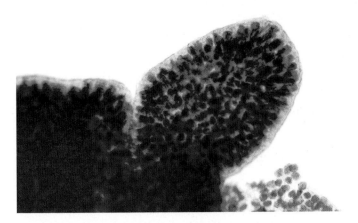

FIGURE 8.25. Papillary thyroid carcinoma, columnar cell variant of PTC. A crowded, pseudopapillary fragment of columnar tumor cells (ThinPrep, Papanicolaou stain).

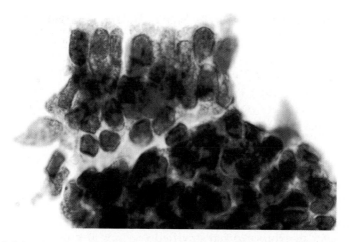

FIGURE 8.26. Papillary thyroid carcinoma, columnar cell variant of PTC. Note the elongated and crowded nuclei with distinct stratification. Cells have dark chromatin, unlike the typical powdery chromatin seen in the other types of PTC (ThinPrep, Papanicolaou stain).

for benign cells like respiratory epithelial cells (seen when the trachea is penetrated). The dark and stratified nuclei resemble those of a colorectal neoplasm, and therefore the possibility of a metastasis from a colorectal primary enters the differential diagnosis. In such cases, an immunocytochemical panel including thyroglobulin, TTF1, and CDX2 can be helpful.

Hyalinizing Trabecular Tumor (Fig. 8.27)

Hyalinizing trabecular tumor (HTT) is a controversial neoplasm that some consider a variant of PTC.

Definition

The hyalinizing trabecular tumor (HTT) is a rare tumor of follicular cell origin characterized by trabecular growth, marked intratrabecular hyalinization, and the nuclear changes of PTC.

Criteria

Cohesive neoplastic cells are radially oriented around amyloid-like hyaline stromal material.
    INCIs and nuclear grooves are numerous.
    Occasional psammoma bodies may be present.
    Cytoplasmic paranuclear yellow bodies may be present.

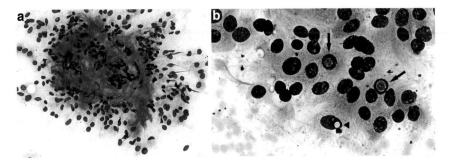

Figure 8.27. Hyalinizing trabecular tumor. (**a**) There is a core of metachromatic hyaline material insinuating among cells with oval nuclei, anisonucleosis, and abundant cytoplasm (smear, Diff-Quik stain). (**b**) Oval neoplastic nuclei have occasional intranuclear cytoplasmic pseudoinclusions (INCIs, *arrows*). Note the clear hole in one of the adjacent nuclei (*arrowhead*), a mimic of INCIs, but recognizable as an artifact because the hole is white rather than the color and texture of cytoplasm (smear, Papanicolaou stain).

Explanatory Notes

The morphologic features of HTT overlap significantly with those of PTC.[35,36] Currently, there is disagreement as to whether this tumor should be considered a variant of PTC or a form of follicular adenoma. The majority behave in a benign fashion, but malignant HTTs have been reported. HTT is very difficult to recognize as such in an FNA specimen. Because of its nuclear features, most HTTs are interpreted as PTC or "suspicious for PTC."

Other Rare Variants

Other histologic variants (e.g., solid, cribriform-morular, diffuse sclerosing) of PTC exist, but their FNA cytologic features have been only very rarely described. Most are difficult if not impossible to distinguish from a conventional PTC by FNA.

Management

Surgical consultation is recommended for patients with an FNA interpretation that is conclusive for PTC. The decision to perform surgery and the extent of surgery (lobectomy vs. total thyroidectomy) that is recommended depend on the patient's age and overall health status and the sonographic characteristics of the malignant nodule. The American Thyroid Association recommends total or near total thyroidectomy if any of the following is present: the malignant nodule is more than 1–1.5 cm, contralateral thyroid nodules, regional or distant metastases, patient has a personal history of radiation therapy to the head and neck, or a first degree family history of differentiated thyroid cancer.[37]

Older age (>45 years) may also be a criterion for recommending near-total or total thyroidectomy because of higher recurrence rates in this age group.

Sample Reports

The general category "MALIGNANT" is used whenever the cytomorphologic features are conclusive for malignancy. If an aspirate is interpreted as malignant, it is implied that the sample is adequate for evaluation. (An explicit statement of adequacy is optional.) Descriptive comments that follow are used to subclassify the malignancy and summarize the results of special studies, if any. If the findings are suspicious but not conclusive for malignancy, the general category "SUSPICIOUS FOR MALIGNANCY" should be used (see Chap. 7).

Example 1
    MALIGNANT.
    Papillary thyroid carcinoma.

Example 2
    MALIGNANT.
    Papillary thyroid carcinoma, favor tall cell variant.

References

1. LiVolsi VA, Albores-Saavedra J, Asa SL. Papillary carcinoma. In: Lellis D, Lloyd R, Heitz PU, Eng C, eds. *WHO classification of tumours. Pathology and genetics of tumours of endocrine organs.* Lyon: IARC Press; 2004:57-66.
2. Yassa L, Cibas ES, Benson CB, et al. Long-term assessment of a multidisciplinary approach to thyroid nodule diagnostic evaluation. *Cancer.* 2007;111(6):508-516.
3. Yang J, Schnadig V, Logrono R, Wasserman PG. Fine-needle aspiration of thyroid nodules: a study of 4703 patients with histologic and clinical correlations. *Cancer.* 2007;111(5):306-315.
4. Gharib H, Goellner JR, Johnson DA. Fine-needle aspiration cytology of the thyroid: a 12-year experience with 11, 000 biopsies. *Clin Lab Med.* 1993;13:699-709.
5. Wang HH. Reporting thyroid fine-needle aspiration: literature review and a proposal. *Diagn Cytopathol.* 2006;34(1):67-76.
6. Renshaw AA. Accuracy of thyroid fine-needle aspiration using receiver operator characteristic curves. *Am J Clin Pathol.* 2001;116:477-482.
7. Baloch ZW, LiVolsi VA. Fine-needle aspiration of thyroid nodules: past, present, and future. *Endocr Pract.* 2004;10(3):234-241.
8. Miller TR, Bottles K, Holly EA, Friend NF, Abele JS. A step-wise logistic regression analysis of papillary carcinoma of the thyroid. *Acta Cytol.* 1986;30(3):285-293.
9. Kini SR. *Thyroid cytopathology: An atlas and text.* Philadelphia: Lippincott Williams & Wilkins; 2008.
10. Lloyd RV, Erickson LA, Casey MB, et al. Observer variation in the diagnosis of follicular variant of papillary thyroid carcinoma. *Am J Surg Pathol.* 2004;28(10):1336-1340.

11. Renshaw AA. How closely do thyroid fine-needle aspirates need to be screened? *Diagn Cytopathol.* 2002;27(5):259-260.

12. Renshaw AA. Focal features of papillary carcinoma of the thyroid in fine-needle aspiration material are strongly associated with papillary carcinoma at resection. *Am J Clin Pathol.* 2002;118(2):208-210.

13. Hirokawa M, Carney JA, Goellner JR, et al. Observer variation of encapsulated follicular lesions of the thyroid gland. *Am J Surg Pathol.* 2002;26(11):1508-1514.

14. Baloch ZW, Livolsi VA. Follicular-patterned lesions of the thyroid: the bane of the pathologist. *Am J Clin Pathol.* 2002;117(1):143-150.

15. Renshaw AA, Gould EW. Why there is the tendency to "overdiagnose" the follicular variant of papillary thyroid carcinoma. *Am J Clin Pathol.* 2002;117(1):19-21.

16. Renshaw AA. "Histiocytoid" cells in fine-needle aspirations of papillary carcinoma of the thyroid: frequency and significance of an under-recognized cytologic pattern. *Cancer.* 2002;96(4):240-243.

17. Rupp M, Ehya H. Nuclear grooves in the aspiration cytology of papillary carcinoma of the thyroid. *Acta Cytol.* 1989;33(1):21-26.

18. Papotti M, Manazza AD, Chiarle R, Bussolati G. Confocal microscope analysis and tridimensional reconstruction of papillary thyroid carcinoma nuclei. *Virchows Arch.* 2004;444(4):350-355.

19. Ellison E, Lapuerta P, Martin SE. Psammoma bodies in fine-needle aspirates of the thyroid: predictive value for papillary carcinoma. *Cancer.* 1998;84(3):169-175.

20. Rosai J, Zampi G, Carcangiu ML. Papillary carcinoma of the thyroid. A discussion of its several morphologic expressions, with particular emphasis on the follicular variant. *Am J Surg Pathol.* 1983;7(8):809-817.

21. Carcangiu ML, Zampi G, Pupi A, Castagnoli A, Rosai J. Papillary carcinoma of the thyroid. A clinicopathologic study of 241 cases treated at the University of Florence, Italy. *Cancer.* 1985;55(4):805-828.

22. Baloch ZW, Gupta PK, Yu GH, Sack MJ, LiVolsi VA. Follicular variant of papillary carcinoma. Cytologic and histologic correlation. *Am J Clin Pathol.* 1999;111(2):216-222.

23. Fulciniti F, Benincasa G, Vetrani A, Palombini L. Follicular variant of papillary carcinoma: cytologic findings on FNAB samples-experience with 16 cases. *Diagn Cytopathol.* 2001;25(2):86-93.

24. Goodell WM, Saboorian MH, Ashfaq R. Fine-needle aspiration diagnosis of the follicular variant of papillary carcinoma. *Cancer.* 1998;84(6):349-354.

25. Mesonero CE, Jugle JE, Wilbur DC, Nayar R. Fine-needle aspiration of the macrofollicular and microfollicular subtypes of the follicular variant of papillary carcinoma of the thyroid. *Cancer.* 1998;84(4):235-244.

26. Chung D, Ghossein RA, Lin O. Macrofollicular variant of papillary carcinoma: a potential thyroid FNA pitfall. *Diagn Cytopathol.* 2007;35(9):560-564.

27. Goellner JR, Johnson DA. Cytology of cystic papillary carcinoma of the thyroid. *Acta Cytol.* 1982;26(6):797-808.

28. Faquin WC, Cibas ES, Renshaw AA. "Atypical" cells in fine-needle aspiration biopsy specimens of benign thyroid cysts. *Cancer.* 2005;105(2):71-79.

29. Moreira AL, Waisman J, Cangiarella JF. Aspiration cytology of the oncocytic variant of papillary adenocarcinoma of the thyroid gland. *Acta Cytol.* 2004;48(2):137-141.

30. Doria MI Jr, Attal H, Wang HH, Jensen JA, DeMay RM. Fine needle aspiration cytology of the oxyphil variant of papillary carcinoma of the thyroid. A report of three cases. *Acta Cytol.* 1996;40(5):1007-1011.

31. Baloch ZW, LiVolsi VA. Warthin-like papillary carcinoma of the thyroid. *Arch Pathol Lab Med.* 2000;124(8):1192-1195.

32. Ghossein RA, LiVolsi VA. Papillary carcinoma, tall cell variant. *Thyroid*. 2008;18(11):1179-1181.
33. Solomon A, Gupta PK, LiVolsi VA, Baloch ZW. Distinguishing tall cell variant of papillary thyroid carcinoma from usual variant of papillary thyroid carcinoma in cytologic specimens. *Diagn Cytopathol*. 2002;27(3):143-148.
34. Jayaram G. Cytology of columnar-cell variant of papillary thyroid carcinoma. *Diagn Cytopathol*. 2000;22(4):227-229.
35. Goellner JR, Carney JA. Cytologic features of fine needle aspirates of hyalinizing trabecular adenoma of the thyroid. *Am J Clin Pathol*. 1989;91:115-119.
36. Casey MB, Sebo TJ, Carney JA. Hyalinizing trabecular adenoma of the thyroid gland: cytologic features in 29 cases. *Am J Surg Pathol*. 2004;28(7):859-867.
37. Cooper DS, Doherty GM, Haugen BR, et al. Management guidelines for patients with thyroid nodules and differentiated thyroid cancer. *Thyroid*. 2006;16(2):109-142.

Chapter 9

Medullary Thyroid Carcinoma

Martha B. Pitman, Yolanda C. Oertel, and Kim R. Geisinger

Background

In 1951 Horn described and illustrated what is now known as medullary thyroid carcinoma (MTC).[1] A few years later, Hazard and colleagues reported 21 cases of "this medullary or solid form of thyroid carcinoma" and recommended that it be recognized as a distinct clinicopathologic entity.[2] In 1966, Williams suggested that it was derived from the calcitonin-producing "C cells" or parafollicular cells of the thyroid.[3] A few years later, investigators showed conclusively that MTCs were immunoreactive for calcitonin.[4,5]

MTC comprises approximately 7% of thyroid carcinomas. It occurs in sporadic (in 85% of cases) and heritable forms. The heritable forms include multiple endocrine neoplasia (MEN) type 2A (Sipple's syndrome), which includes pheochromocytomas and hyperparathyroidism in some families; MEN type 2B (mucosal neuroma syndrome or Gorlin's syndrome), which consistently includes mucosal neuromas and somatic marfanoid habitus; and familial medullary thyroid carcinoma (FMTC). The hereditary forms are characterized by an autosomal dominant mode of inheritance and are associated with point mutations in the *RET* proto-oncogene on chromosome 10.

MTC may occur at any age, including infancy. Patients with FMTC and sporadic tumors, however, are usually older adults with a mean age of 50 years. MTC is an aggressive tumor that spreads by hematogenous and lymphatic routes. Common sites of metastasis include cervical lymph nodes, lung, liver, bone, and adrenal glands. Up to 50% of patients present with cervical nodal metastases, and in these patients the primary tumor can be occult.[6] For this reason, the possibility of metastatic MTC should be kept in mind in a patient with a positive cervical lymph node of unknown primary.

Some generalizations can be made about the usual histologic and cytologic appearance of MTCs, but this tumor has a large number of variants: papillary (or pseudopapillary); glandular; giant cell; spindle cell; small cell and

Syed Z. Ali and Edmund S. Cibas (eds.), *The Bethesda System for Reporting*
Thyroid Cytopathology, DOI 10.1007/ 978-0-387-87666-5_9,
© Springer Science+Business Media, LLC 2010

neuroblastoma-like; paraganglioma-like; oncocytic; clear cell; angiosarcoma-like; squamous cell; melanin-producing; and amphicrine.[6] This morphologic heterogeneity leads to significant diagnostic challenges in the histologic and cytologic evaluation of this neoplasm.

Definition

MTC is a malignant neoplasm derived from and/or morphologically recapitulating the parafollicular cells of the thyroid gland.

Criteria (Figs. 9.1–9.16)

Samples show moderate to marked cellularity.

Numerous isolated cells alternate with syncytial-like clusters in variable proportions from case to case.

Cells are plasmacytoid, polygonal, round, and/or spindle-shaped. Long cell processes are seen in some cases.

The neoplastic cells usually show only mild to moderate pleomorphism.

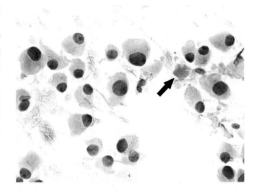

FIGURE 9.1. Medullary thyroid carcinoma. Predominantly dispersed, uniform plasmacytoid or polygonal cells have granular ("salt and pepper") chromatin and small but distinct nucleoli. A small fragment of amyloid is present (arrow). This tumor presented as a cervical node metastasis, a common clinical presentation (smear, Papanicolaou stain).

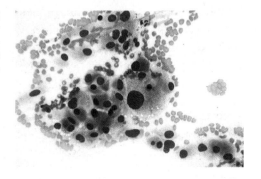

FIGURE 9.2. Medullary thyroid carcinoma. Variation in nuclear size and shape, typical of neuroendocrine tumors in general, is common in medullary thyroid carcinoma (smear, Diff-Quik stain).

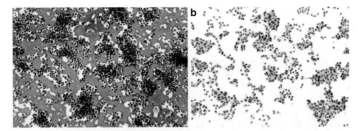

Figure 9.3. Medullary thyroid carcinoma. A combination of anastomosing syncytial-like clusters, trabeculae, and isolated cells is in keeping with a neuroendocrine tumor. Most of the nuclei are round, with mild pleomorphism. Cytoplasm is basophilic and moderate in volume (smears: A. Diff-Quik stain; B. Papanicolaou stain).

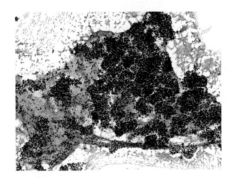

Figure 9.4. Medullary thyroid carcinoma. A smear pattern in which cohesive, syncytial-like clusters predominate, with few isolated cells, thus mimicking a follicular neoplasm or poorly differentiated carcinoma, is occasionally encountered (smear, Papanicolaou stain).

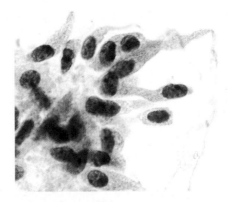

Figure 9.5. Medullary thyroid carcinoma. A spindle-cell pattern predominates in some tumors. Note the elongated cells with abundant granular cytoplasm and long cytoplasmic processes. The coarsely textured chromatin typical of medullary thyroid carcinomas is apparent (ThinPrep, Papanicolaou stain).

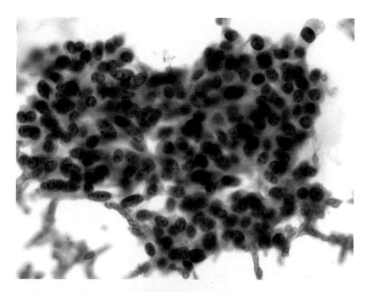

FIGURE 9.6. Medullary thyroid carcinoma. Syncytial-like clusters of tumor cells are variable in size and shape. The uniformity of the cells, coarse chromatin, absence of prominent nucleoli, and scant cytoplasm are apparent (smear, Papanicolaou stain).

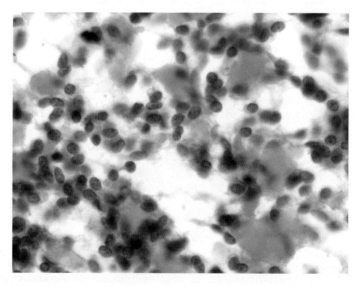

FIGURE 9.7. Medullary thyroid carcinoma. Amyloid is abundant and readily appreciated in some cases (smear, Papanicolaou stain).

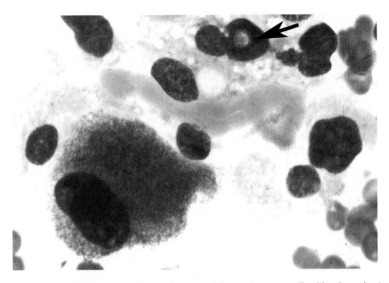

FIGURE 9.8. Medullary thyroid carcinoma. A large tumor cell with abundant cytoplasm displays red cytoplasmic granules with a Romanowsky-type stain. Note also the presence of amyloid, one neoplastic cell with an intranuclear pseudoinclusion (arrow), and scattered bare nuclei of tumor cells (smear, Diff-Quik stain).

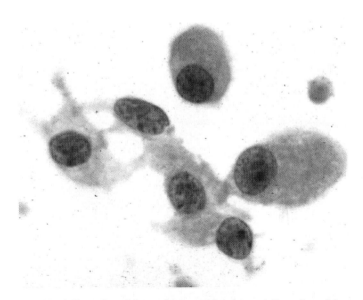

FIGURE 9.9. Medullary thyroid carcinoma. Many medullary thyroid carcinoma cells have a plasmacytoid appearance, considered the classic pattern of this tumor. The cells have a round nucleus, eccentrically placed within a moderately abundant, granular cytoplasm that stains green-blue with the Papanicolaou stain. Some cells have small nucleoli (smear, Papanicolaou stain).

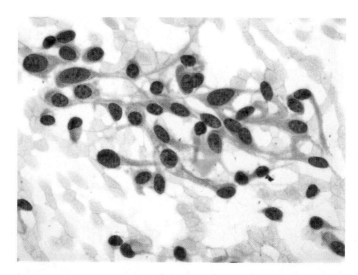

FIGURE 9.10. Medullary thyroid carcinoma. The spindle cell variant has prominent interdigitating cytoplasmic processes with oval nuclei. Smooth nuclear membranes, coarse chromatin, and inconspicuous nucleoli are maintained (smear, Papanicolaou stain).

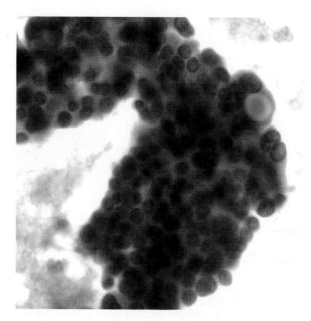

FIGURE 9.11. Medullary thyroid carcinoma. Cytoplasmic vacuoles can occasionally be seen in medullary carcinoma (smear, Papanicolaou stain).

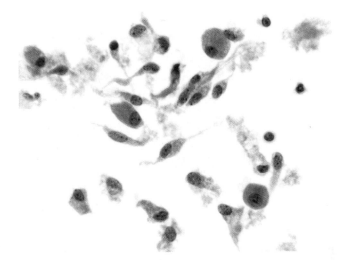

FIGURE 9.12. Medullary thyroid carcinoma. A variety of shapes (round, polygonal, plasmacytoid, and spindled) are noted in this non-cohesive population of tumor cells processed by a liquid-based method (ThinPrep, Papanicolaou stain).

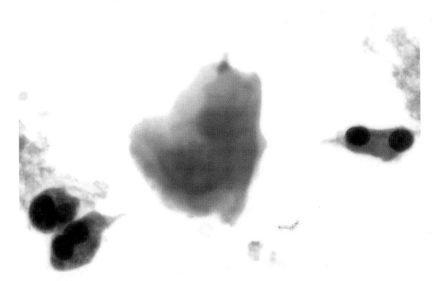

FIGURE 9.13. Medullary thyroid carcinoma. Amyloid has the same dense, amorphous, waxy appearance on liquid-based preparations as it does on smears (ThinPrep, Papanicolaou stain).

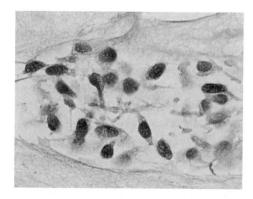

FIGURE 9.14. Medullary thyroid carcinoma. The needle rinse sample can be processed as a cell block. Morphologic features mimic those seen on smears and liquid-based preparations. Here the elongated cells have an oval nucleus with coarsely granular chromatin and elongated pink, granular cytoplasm (cell block, hematoxylin and eosin stain).

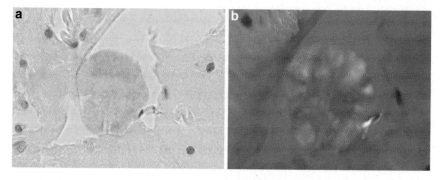

FIGURE 9.15. Medullary thyroid carcinoma. (a) Amyloid stains orange-red with the Congo red stain. (b) Under polarized light, the Congo red stain turns an apple-green color. (a, b. Cell block, Congo red stain).

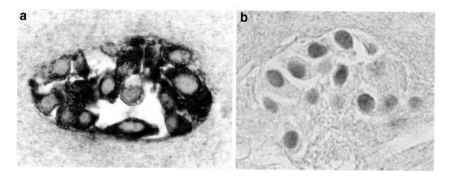

FIGURE 9.16. Medullary thyroid carcinoma. (a). The tumor cells are immunoreactive for calcitonin. (b). They are negative for thyroglobulin. (a, b. Cell block preparations, hematoxylin counterstain).

Rare bizarre giant cells may be seen; they can be numerous in the giant cell variant.

Nuclei are round and often eccentrically placed, with finely or coarsely granular ("salt and pepper") chromatin.

Nuclear pseudoinclusions are occasionally noted.

Binucleation and multinucleation are common.

Nucleoli are usually inconspicuous but can be prominent in some cells.

Cytoplasm is granular and variable in quantity. Small red granules are seen with Romanowsky stains in some cases. Rare cases show cytoplasmic melanin pigment.

Amyloid is often present and appears as dense, amorphous material that resembles thick colloid.

Cells are typically strongly immunoreactive for calcitonin, CEA, chromogranin, synaptophysin, and TTF-1, and are negative for thyroglobulin. (Aberrant results occasionally occur).

Explanatory Notes

Cytologic preparations from a MTC are usually moderately or highly cellular and composed of a mixture of non-cohesive cells and cell aggregates.[7–10] The proportion of isolated cells versus aggregates varies from case to case.[8,11] Tumor cell aggregates vary in size and may have a syncytial-like appearance because cell membranes are indistinct. Bare nuclei and nuclear molding are seen in some cases.[11] In most cases, the majority of the neoplastic cells are uniform in appearance, with only mild to moderate pleomorphism,[8,11,12] but occasional cases show marked pleomorphism.[12] Intranuclear pseudoinclusions (indistinguishable from those seen in papillary carcinoma) are encountered in one-half of cases.[12,13] The characteristic red granules seen with Romanowsky stains are not found in all cases of MTC; when present, they are usually found in the larger or multinucleated cells.[8,11,13] Estimates of the frequency of amyloid vary from almost one-half to 80% of cases.[8,11–13] Amyloid can be intermixed with tumor cells or separated from them.[7]

The diagnosis of MTC can be strongly suggested by cytomorphology alone, but it is advisable to confirm the interpretation with a Congo red stain for amyloid and/or immunohistochemical studies. A panel of immunohistochemical stains, including some stains that are expected to be positive (e.g., calcitonin, CEA, chromogranin, and synaptophysin) and others expected to be negative (e.g., thyroglobulin) is preferable to solitary antibody staining, because aberrant results can occur with any given antibody. Occasional MTCs are negative for calcitonin; conversely, false-positive staining for thyroglobulin has been observed. Cell blocks are the ideal material for immunohistochemistry.

Cytospins, direct smears, and liquid-based preparations can also be used, but protocols should be validated.[14] If histochemical and immunohistochemical confirmation is not possible due to limited material, blood calcitonin levels can be helpful, because most patients with MTC have elevated serum calcitonin levels (≥10 pg ml).[14]

The tumor most commonly confused with MTC is a Hürthle cell neoplasm, but papillary carcinoma, anaplastic carcinoma, hyalinizing trabecular tumor (HTT), plasmacytoma,[15] and metastatic tumors (particularly melanoma) warrant consideration in some instances. The monomorphic appearance, granular cytoplasm, and often eccentric nucleus of Hürthle cell neoplasms mimic MTC cells (see Fig. 6.12a), but smooth, finely textured chromatin and prominent macronucleoli help to identify Hürthle cell neoplasms correctly (see Figs. 6.5 and 6.7). With Romanowsky stains, the cytoplasmic granules of Hürthle cell neoplasms stain blue, not red. Intranuclear pseudoinclusions (cytoplasmic invaginations), so typical of papillary carcinoma, are occasionally noted in MTCs, but papillary architecture, dense (rather than granular) cytoplasm, powdery (rather than coarse) chromatin, and positive immunoreactivity for thyroglobulin help to identify papillary carcinoma and distinguish it from MTC. The spindle cell variant of MTC introduces anaplastic carcinoma, the very rare nodular fasciitis-like variant of papillary carcinoma, and metastatic melanoma into the differential diagnosis. MTC and HTT have overlapping morphologic features and might be mistaken for each other: the stromal component of a HTT resembles amyloid, and both may be composed predominantly of non-cohesive cells with occasional nuclear pseudoinclusions (see Fig. 8.27b). Immunohistochemistry for calcitonin, thyroglobulin, and other markers will usually differentiate MTC from these mimickers.

Management

Surgical treatment of MTC is usually total extracapsular thyroidectomy with lymph node dissection.[16,17] There is no effective treatment currently for recurrent or metastatic disease. Targeted therapy against the *RET* kinase pathway is promising but still investigational.[18]

Sample Reports

The general category "MALIGNANT" is used whenever the cytomorphologic features are conclusive for malignancy. If an aspirate is interpreted as MALIGNANT, it is implied that the sample is adequate for evaluation. (An explicit statement of adequacy is optional.) Descriptive comments that follow are used to subclassify the malignancy and summarize the results of special studies, if any. If the findings are suspicious but not conclusive for malignancy, the general category "SUSPICIOUS FOR MALIGNANCY" should be used (see Chap. 7).

Example 1:
    MALIGNANT.
    Medullary thyroid carcinoma.
    Note: A Congo red stain is positive for amyloid. Immunohistochemistry performed on cell block/cytocentrifuge/liquid-based preparations (choose one) shows that the malignant cells are immunoreactive for calcitonin, CEA, chromogranin, and TTF-1, and negative for thyroglobulin.

Example 2:
    MALIGNANT.
    Consistent with medullary thyroid carcinoma.
    Note: Cytomorphologic features are characteristic of medullary thyroid carcinoma, but tissue is insufficient for confirmatory immunohistochemical studies. Serum chemistries for calcitonin and CEA might be helpful.

References

1. Horn RC. Carcinoma of the thyroid. Description of a distinctive morphological variant and report of 7 cases. *Cancer* 1951;4:697-707.
2. Hazard JB, Hawk WA, Crile G Jr. Medullary (solid) carcinoma of the thyroid; a clinicopathologic entity. *J Clin Endocrinol Metab.* 1959;19(1):152-161.
3. Williams ED. Histogenesis of medullary carcinoma of the thyroid. *J Clin Pathol.* 1966;19(2):114-118.
4. Bussolati G, Foster GV, Clark MB, et al. Immunofluorescent localisation of calcitonin in medullary C-cell thyroid carcinoma, using antibody to the pure porcine hormone. *Virchows Arch B Cell Pathol.* 1969;2(3):234-238.
5. Meyer JS, Abdel-Bari W. Granules and thyrocalcitonin-like activity in medullary carcinoma of the thyroid gland. *N Engl J Med.* 1968;278(10):523-529.
6. Matias-Guiu X, DeLellis R, Moley JF, et al. Medullary thyroid carcinoma. In: DeLellis RA, Lloyd RV, Heitz PU, Eng C, eds. *World Health Organization Classification of Tumours Pathology and Genetics of Endocrine Organs.* Lyon: IARC Press; 2004:86-91.
7. Baloch ZW, LiVolsi VA, Asa SL, et al. Diagnostic terminology and morphologic criteria for cytologic diagnosis of thyroid lesions: a synopsis of the National Cancer Institute Thyroid Fine-Needle Aspiration State of the Science Conference. *Diagn Cytopathol.* 2008;36(6):425-437.
8. Forrest CH, Frost FA, de Boer WB, et al. Medullary carcinoma of the thyroid: accuracy of diagnosis of fine-needle aspiration cytology. *Cancer.* 1998;84(5):295-302.
9. Hsieh MH, Hsiao YL, Chang TC. Fine needle aspiration cytology stained with Rius method in quicker diagnosis of medullary thyroid carcinoma. *J Formos Med Assoc.* 2007;106(9):728-735.

10. Collins BT, Cramer HM, Tabatowski K, et al. Fine needle aspiration of medullary carcinoma of the thyroid. Cytomorphology, immunocytochemistry and electron microscopy. *Acta Cytol* 1995;39(5):920-930.
11. Green I, Ali SZ, Allen EA, et al. A spectrum of cytomorphologic variations in medullary thyroid carcinoma. Fine-needle aspiration findings in 19 cases. *Cancer* 1997;81(1): 40–44.
12. Bose S, Kapila K, Verma K. Medullary carcinoma of the thyroid: a cytological, immunocytochemical, and ultrastructural study. *Diagn Cytopathol.* 1992;8(1):28-32.
13. Us-Krasovec M, Auersperg M, Bergant D, et al. Medullary carcinoma of the thyroid gland: diagnostic cytopathologic characteristics. *Pathologica.* 1998;90:5-13.
14. Filie AC, Asa SL, Geisinger KR, et al. Utilization of ancillary studies in thyroid fine needle aspirates: a synopsis of the National Cancer Institute Thyroid Fine Needle Aspiration State of the Science Conference. *Diagn Cytopathol.* 2008;36(6):438-441.
15. Bourtsos EP, Bedrossian CW, De Frias DV, et al. Thyroid plasmacytoma mimicking medullary carcinoma: a potential pitfall in aspiration cytology. *Diagn Cytopathol.* 2000;23(5):354-358.
16. Layfield L, Cochand-Priollet B, LiVolsi V, et al. Post Thyroid FNA Testing and Treatment Options: a Synopsis of the National Cancer Institute Thyroid Fine Needle Aspiration State of the Science Conference. *Diagn Cytopathol.* 2008;36(6):442-448.
17. Jimenez C, Hu MI, Gagel RF. Management of medullary thyroid carcinoma. *Endocrinol Metab Clin North Am* 2008;37(2):481–496, x-xi.
18. Hong D, Ye L, Gagel R, et al. Medullary thyroid cancer: targeting the RET kinase pathway with sorafenib/tipifarnib. *Mol Cancer Ther.* 2008;7(5):1001-1006.

Chapter 10

Poorly Differentiated Thyroid Carcinoma

Massimo Bongiovanni and William C. Faquin

Background

Poorly differentiated thyroid carcinoma (PDTC) was first proposed as a distinct subtype of thyroid malignancy by Carcangiu et al.[1] These authors reinterpreted the original observation made in 1907 by Langhans, who described a locally aggressive tumor with a peculiar architecture: tumor cells arranged in large, round to oval formations, the so-called "insulae."[2] Currently, there are 2 recognized subtypes of PDTC - insular and non-insular.[3] PDTC is a rare malignancy, accounting for 4–7% of all thyroid cancers.[3] It has an aggressive clinical behavior intermediate between that of the well differentiated thyroid carcinomas (papillary carcinoma, follicular carcinoma, and Hürthle cell carcinoma) and undifferentiated (anaplastic) thyroid carcinoma. PDTCs often present at an advanced stage, have a propensity for local recurrence, and tend to metastasize to regional lymph nodes, lung, and bones. The mean 5-year survival of patients with PDTC is approximately 50%.[3,4] Well differentiated thyroid carcinomas with a focal (10% or greater) PDTC component follow a more aggressive clinical course than standard well differentiated carcinomas of the thyroid.[5]

Definition

PDTC is a thyroid carcinoma of follicular cell origin characterized by an insular, solid, or trabecular growth pattern. In its pure form, PDTC lacks conventional nuclear features of papillary thyroid carcinoma and is distinguished from the latter by the presence of poorly differentiated features: mitoses, necrosis, or small convoluted nuclei. The most classic form of PDTC is the insular type, defined by its "cellular nests" or insular cell groups outlined by a thin fibrovascular border. In a subset of cases, PDTCs can also

Syed Z. Ali and Edmund S. Cibas (eds.), *The Bethesda System for Reporting Thyroid Cytopathology*, DOI 10.1007/ 978-0-387-87666-5_10,
© Springer Science+Business Media, LLC 2010

be associated with a better differentiated component showing typical microscopic features of papillary or follicular carcinoma variably admixed with poorly differentiated cells.

Criteria (Figs. 10.1–10.12)

Cellular preparations display an insular, solid, or trabecular cytoarchitecture (Figs. 10.1–10.4).

There is a uniform population of follicular cells with scant cytoplasm (sometimes plasmacytoid) (Fig. 10.5).

The malignant cells have a high nuclear/cytoplasmic (N/C) ratio with variable nuclear atypia (Figs. 10.6–10.7).

Apoptosis and mitotic activity are present (Fig. 10.8).

Necrosis is often present (Fig. 10.9).

Explanatory Notes

Cytologically, PDTCs are difficult to recognize as such because they are rare; their cytomorphologic features overlap with those of follicular neoplasms; and their characteristic FNA features do not have great specificity.

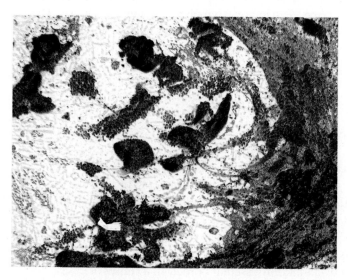

FIGURE 10.1. Poorly differentiated thyroid carcinoma. A low magnification view reveals small follicular cells arranged in crowded insulae. (smear, Papanicolaou stain).

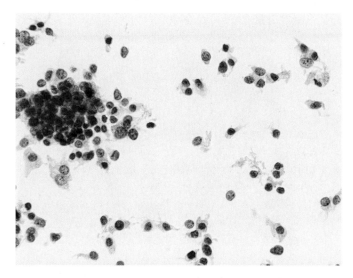

Figure 10.2. Poorly differentiated thyroid carcinoma. The monomorphic cells are arranged in crowded 3-dimensional groups and scattered as isolated cells (ThinPrep, Papanicolaou stain).

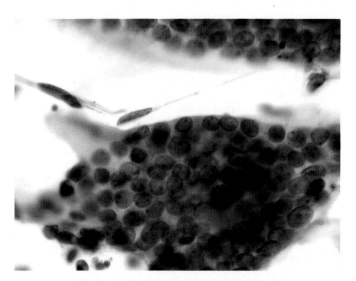

Figure 10.3. Poorly differentiated thyroid carcinoma. Endothelium wrapping around cell groups can often be found highlighting the insular arrangements (smear, Papanicolaou stain).

Based upon a limited number of published case reports and small series, aspirates of PDTC are often cellular with scant colloid.[6–13] The follicular cells of PDTC have a monomorphic appearance at low magnification owing to their high N/C ratio and round nuclei, but at higher magnification

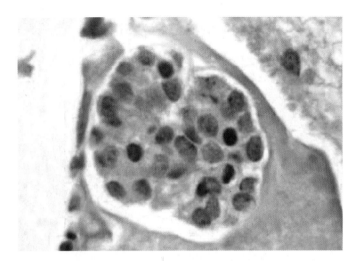

Figure 10.4. Poorly differentiated thyroid carcinoma. This cell block demonstrates the arrangement of cells in insular groups (cell block, H&E stain).

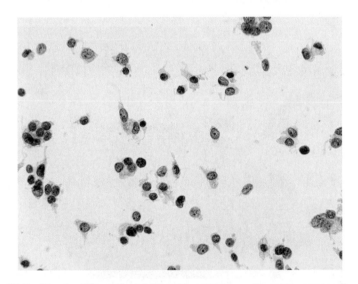

Figure 10.5. Poorly differentiated thyroid carcinoma. In some cases, the malignant cells are arranged predominantly as isolated cells. They can have a plasmacytoid cytomorphology, as seen here (ThinPrep, Papanicolaou stain).

variable degrees of atypia can be found. Numerous isolated cells alternate with large solid fragments of mitotically active and apoptotic cells. The proportion of isolated cells versus fragments varies from case to case. Necrosis is often seen.

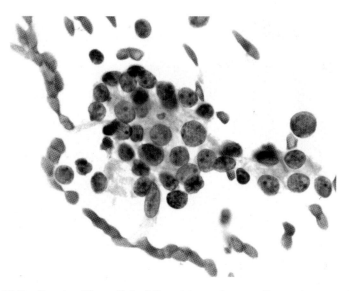

Figure 10.6. Poorly differentiated thyroid carcinoma. Some tumors demonstrate only mild nuclear atypia, with small nucleoli and delicate chromatin (smear, Papanicolaou stain).

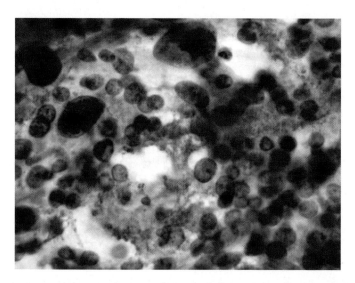

Figure 10.7. Poorly differentiated thyroid carcinoma. Some aspirates exhibit marked nuclear atypia. In this example, there is impressive anisokaryosis (smear, Papanicolaou stain).

The insular form of PDTC is identified histologically by its characteristic arrangement of cells in insulae with peripheral endothelial wrapping. A similar pattern can be recognized in a subset of PDTC aspirates.

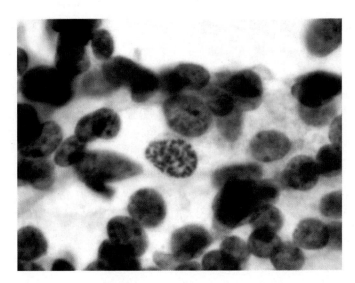

FIGURE **10.8.** Poorly differentiated thyroid carcinoma. Aspirates of poorly differentiated carcinomas will often contain mitotically active cells (smear, Papanicolaou stain).

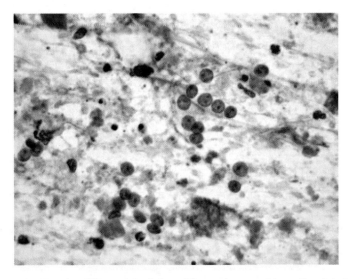

FIGURE **10.9.** Poorly differentiated thyroid carcinoma. Necrotic debris (cytoplasmic and nuclear fragments) is seen in some poorly differentiated carcinomas (smear, Papanicolaou stain).

Depending upon whether a well differentiated component is also present, aspirates of PDTC can exhibit microfollicles, nuclear grooves, and pseudoinclusions (Figure 10.10). In the majority of cases, PDTCs are diagnosed cytologically as "Suspicious for a Follicular Neoplasm." In the largest series

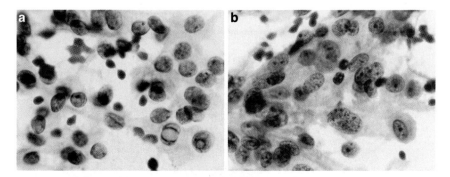

FIGURE **10.10.** Poorly differentiated thyroid carcinoma. (**a**). In some areas, this tumor showed features of papillary carcinoma, including nuclear grooves and pseudoinclusions. (**b**). In other areas, the tumor cells showed significant nuclear pleomorphism. (**a** and **b**, smears, Papanicolaou stain).

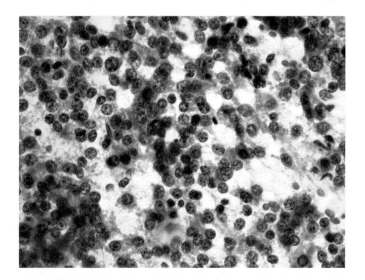

FIGURE **10.11.** Poorly differentiated thyroid carcinoma. Because some aspirates are comprised predominantly of isolated cells with granular chromatin, they can mimic both a medullary thyroid carcinoma and a metastatic neoplasm (smear, Papanicolaou stain).

of PDTCs sampled by FNA (40 cases), only 13 (32.5%) were prospectively recognized as "poorly differentiated carcinoma" by FNA.[14] The other cases were diagnosed as "carcinoma, not otherwise specified" (10%), papillary carcinoma (15%), and "suspicious for a follicular neoplasm" (42.5%). Using logistic regression analysis, the features most predictive of PDTC were its

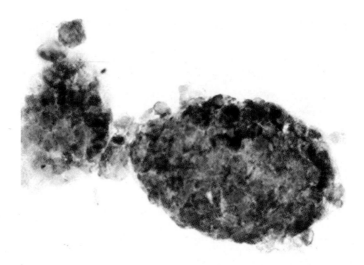

FIGURE **10.12.** Poorly differentiated thyroid carcinoma. Poorly differentiated thyroid carcinomas are positive for thyroglobulin, which helps to distinguish them from medullary carcinoma and metastatic tumors (ThinPrep, thyroglobulin immunohistochemical reaction).

characteristic cytoarchitecture (neither macrofollicular nor microfollicular), severe crowding, high N/C ratio, and isolated cells.[14]

According to the authors of the WHO volume on Pathology and Genetics of Tumours of Endocrine Organs, "a definitive diagnosis of poorly differentiated carcinoma can be made only at the histological level."[3] The combination of cytomorphologic features described above, however, is suggestive of PDTC in FNA specimens. Clinical and ultrasonographic correlation is also helpful: PDTCs are usually large tumors with extra-thyroidal extension.

Certain other primary thyroid tumors and metastatic malignancy should be considered in the differential diagnosis of a PDTC. A subset of PDTCs exhibits a predominantly isolated-cell pattern in FNA samples (Fig. 10.11). When this occurs, together with a "salt and pepper-like" chromatin pattern, the possibility of medullary thyroid carcinoma should be excluded with immunoperoxidase stains. In contrast to medullary thyroid carcinoma, most PDTCs are strongly immunoreactive for thyroglobulin (Fig. 10.12) and negative for calcitonin and CEA. In addition, PDTCs are rarely immunoreactive for neuroendocrine markers such as synaptophysin and chromogranin. TTF-1 is not useful because both PDTC and medullary thyroid carcinoma are positive. Based purely on cytomorphology, a PDTC resembles a metastasis from an extrathyroidal primary tumor: both yield cellular specimens with nuclear atypia and necrosis, and colloid is scant in both. The positive immunoreactivity of PDTCs for thyroglobulin and TTF-1 helps to exclude a metastasis. Undifferentiated (anaplastic) thyroid carcinomas are also characterized by unusual cytomorphologic patterns (see Chap. 11) together with necrosis and increased mitotic activity, but PDTCs lack the marked nuclear pleomorphism, high-grade atypia, and sarcomatoid features seen in undifferentiated carcinomas. The subset of PDTCs with a predominantly isolated-cell pattern and plasmacytoid cytomorphology can suggest a lymphoproliferative disorder, but PDTCs are negative for CD45, as well as markers of B cells (e.g., CD19, CD20) and plasma cells (e.g., CD138).

Management

Because of their poor clinical prognosis, PDTCs are usually managed more aggressively than well differentiated thyroid carcinomas. A recent evidence-based review of therapeutic options for PDTCs recommends using ^{131}I therapy postoperatively.[15] For stage T3 PDTCs without distant metastases, as well as all T4 tumors and cases with regional lymph node involvement, patients benefit from external beam radiotherapy in addition to surgery.

Sample Reports

The general category "MALIGNANT" is used whenever the cytomorphologic features are conclusive for malignancy. If an aspirate is interpreted as MALIGNANT, it is implied that the sample is adequate for evaluation. (An explicit statement of adequacy is optional). Descriptive comments that follow are used to subclassify the malignancy and summarize the results of special studies, if any. If the findings are suspicious but not conclusive for malignancy, the general category "SUSPICIOUS FOR MALIGNANCY" should be used (see Chap. 7). Many PDTCs overlap morphologically with follicular neoplasms and are therefore inevitably interpreted as "SUSPICIOUS FOR A FOLLICULAR NEOPLASM" (or "FOLLICULAR NEOPLASM").

Example 1:
  MALIGNANT.
  Highly cellular aspirate with atypical follicular cells, necrosis, and scant colloid, most consistent with poorly differentiated thyroid carcinoma.

Example 2:
  MALIGNANT.
  Papillary thyroid carcinoma with poorly differentiated features, suggestive of poorly differentiated thyroid carcinoma.

Example 3:
  SUSPICIOUS FOR A FOLLICULAR NEOPLASM.

Atypical follicular cells with a prominent isolated-cell component, focal necrosis, and mitotic activity.

Note: Immunostains on cell block sections show that the lesional cells are immunoreactive for thyroglobulin and TTF-1 and negative for calcitonin. The findings suggest the possibility of a poorly differentiated thyroid carcinoma.

References

1. Carcangiu ML, Zampi G, Rosai J. Poorly differentiated ("insular") thyroid carcinoma. A reinterpretation of Langhans' "wuchernde struma". Am J Surg Pathol 1984;8(9): 655-668.
2. Langhans T. Uber die epithelialen formen der malignen struma. *Virchows Arch (A)*. 1907;189:69-188.
3. Sobrinho Simoes M, Albores-Saavedra J, Tallini G, et al. Poorly differentiated carcinoma. In: DeLellis R, Lloyd RV, Heitz PU, Eng C, eds. *World Health Organization Classification of Tumours: Pathology and Genetics of Tumours of Endocrine Organs.* Lyon: IARC Press 2004.
4. Volante M, Landolfi S, Chiusa L, et al. Poorly differentiated carcinomas of the thyroid with trabecular, insular, and solid patterns: a clinicopathologic study of 183 patients. *Cancer*. 2004;100(5):950-957.
5. Decaussin M, Bernard MH, Adeleine P, et al. Thyroid carcinomas with distant metastases: a review of 111 cases with emphasis on the prognostic significance of an insular component. *Am J Surg Pathol*. 2002;26(8):1007-1015.
6. Bedrossian CWM, Martinez F, Silverberg AB. Fine needle aspiration. In: Gnepp DR, ed. *Pathology of the head and neck*. New York: Churchill Livingstone; 1988:25-99.
7. Flynn SD, Forman BH, Stewart AF, et al. Poorly differentiated ("insular") carcinoma of the thyroid gland: an aggressive subset of differentiated thyroid neoplasms. *Surgery*. 1988;104(6):963-970.
8. Pietribiasi F, Sapino A, Papotti M, et al. Cytologic features of poorly differentiated 'insular' carcinoma of the thyroid, as revealed by fine-needle aspiration biopsy. *Am J Clin Pathol*. 1990;94:687-692.
9. Sironi M, Collini P, Cantaboni A. Fine needle aspiration cytology of insular thyroid carcinoma: a report of four cases. *Acta Cytol*. 1992;36:435-439.
10. Guiter GE, Auger M, Ali SZ, et al. Cytopathology of insular carcinoma of the thyroid. *Cancer (Cancer Cytopathol)*. 1999;87:196-202.
11. Nguyen GK, Akin M-RM. Cytopathology of insular carcinoma of the thyroid. *Diagn Cytopathol*. 2001;25:325-330.
12. Oertel YC, Miyahara-Felipe L. Cytologic features of insular carcinoma of the thyroid: a case report. *Diagn Cytopathol*. 2006;34(8):572-575.
13. Zakowski MF, Schlesinger K, Mizrachi HH. Cytologic features of poorly differentiated "insular" carcinoma of the thyroid. A case report. *Acta Cytol* 1992;36(4):523-526.
14. Bongiovanni M, Bloom L, Krane JF, et al. Cytomorphologic features of poorly differentiated thyroid carcinoma. A multi-institutional analysis of 40 cases. *Cancer* (Cancer Cytopathol) 2009;117(3):185-194.
15. Sanders EM Jr, LiVolsi VA, Brierley J, et al. An evidence-based review of poorly differentiated thyroid cancer. *World J Surg*. 2007;31(5):934-945.

Chapter 11

Undifferentiated (Anaplastic) Carcinoma and Squamous Cell Carcinoma of the Thyroid

Gregg A. Staerkel, Britt-Marie E. Ljung,
Vinod Shidham, William J. Frable, and Juan Rosai

Undifferentiated (Anaplastic) Thyroid Carcinoma

Background

Undifferentiated (anaplastic) thyroid carcinoma (UTC), also called "giant and spindle cell carcinoma," is an extremely aggressive thyroid malignancy. Accounting for less than 5% of malignant thyroid tumors,[1,2] it carries the poorest prognosis as compared to well differentiated and poorly differentiated thyroid carcinomas.[3] Most patients succumb to their disease within six months to one year of their initial diagnosis, typically as a result of tumor involvement of vital structures within the neck.[1,4] Characteristic clinical features are associated with UTCs. These tumors are rarely seen in individuals below the age of 50 (<10% of cases).[2,4,5] There is a female predominance (2–4:1).[2–6] Patients present with a hard, nodular thyroid gland, and most have a rapidly growing mass. Neck enlargement is due to marked tumor growth, with or without reactive fibrosis, which infiltrates into surrounding extrathyroidal soft tissues of the neck, e.g., muscle, trachea, esophagus, and adjacent skin, cartilage, and bone.[4] Half of the patients with UTC report significant neck compression that can result in dyspnea, dysphasia, hoarseness, and/or pain.[1,4] One-quarter to one-half of patients present with lymphadenopathy and/or distant metastases, most commonly to the lungs.[1,3,5] Finally, a history of long standing goiter[1,3,5] and thyroid function tests indicating euthyroidism (despite extensive thyroid gland destruction)[1,5] are common.

Syed Z. Ali and Edmund S. Cibas (eds.), *The Bethesda System for Reporting Thyroid Cytopathology*, DOI 10.1007/ 978-0-387-87666-5_11,
© Springer Science+Business Media, LLC 2010

Definition

UTC is a high grade, pleomorphic, epithelial-derived malignancy with epithelioid and/or spindle cell features.

Criteria (Figs. 11.1–11.15)

Samples show variable cellularity but are usually moderately to markedly cellular.

Neoplastic cells are arranged as isolated cells and/or in variably sized groups.

Neoplastic cells are epithelioid (round to polygonal) and/or spindle-shaped and range in size from small to giant-sized. "Plasmacytoid" and "rhabdoid" cell shapes are seen.

Nuclei show enlargement, irregularity, pleomorphism, clumping of chromatin with parachromatin clearing, prominent irregular nucleoli, intranuclear inclusions, eccentric nuclear placement, and multinucleation.

Necrosis, extensive inflammation (predominantly neutrophils, "abscess-like") and/or fibrous connective tissue may be present.

Osteoclast-like giant cells (non-neoplastic) are conspicuous in some cases.

Neutrophilic infiltration of tumor cell cytoplasm can be seen.

Mitotic figures are often numerous and abnormal.

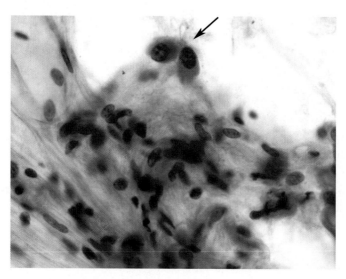

FIGURE 11.1. Undifferentiated (anaplastic) thyroid carcinoma. Aspiration of tumors with abundant fibrosis can yield low cellularity. If cells lack marked nuclear atypia (arrow), rendering a definitive diagnosis can be difficult. Clinical correlation is important (smear, Papanicolaou stain).

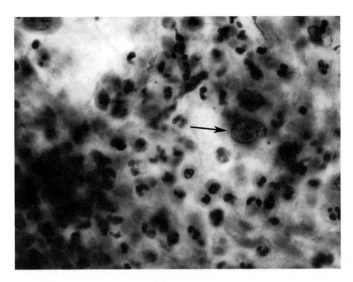

Figure 11.2. Undifferentiated (anaplastic) thyroid carcinoma. Widespread tumor necrosis and associated inflammation can hinder diagnosis because well preserved malignant cells are few and far between (arrow) (smear, Papanicolaou stain).

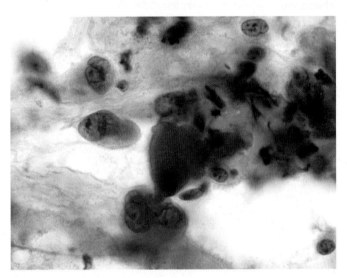

Figure 11.3. Undifferentiated (anaplastic) thyroid carcinoma. Rapid tumor growth and invasion of extrathyroidal tissues is common. Aspiration samples can contain skeletal muscle fragments (center) as well as anaplastic tumor cells (smear, Papanicolaou stain).

Tumors have the following immunochemical profile:

- Pan-keratin and vimentin – positive, often focally (some tumors are negative for one or the other);
- TTF-1 and thyroglobulin – commonly negative

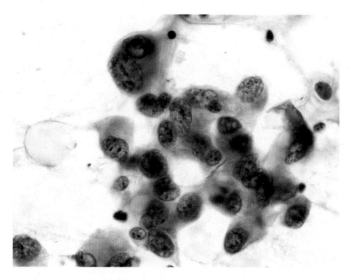

FIGURE 11.4. Undifferentiated (anaplastic) thyroid carcinoma. Cells are epithelioid (polygonal) in appearance. Variation in cell and nuclear size is evident. Parachromatin clearing and nuclear contour irregularity are prominent (smear, Papanicolaou stain).

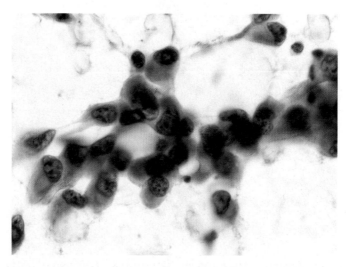

FIGURE 11.5. Undifferentiated (anaplastic) thyroid carcinoma. In some cases, the epithelioid tumor cells have a conspicuously plasmacytoid appearance (smear, Papanicolaou stain).

Explanatory Notes

Cellularity is variable. Some specimens can be sparsely cellular, due in part to the marked fibrosis and hyalinization seen in some tumors.[6-8] When fibrosis predominates, the resulting low cellularity can hamper interpretation.

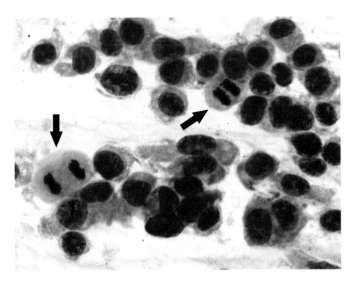

FIGURE 11.6. Undifferentiated (anaplastic) thyroid carcinoma. The neoplastic cells are mostly round, with scant to moderate cytoplasm. There is less pleomorphism of nuclear size and shape than in most cases of UTC, but mitotic figures (arrows) are easily found (smear, Diff-Quik stain).

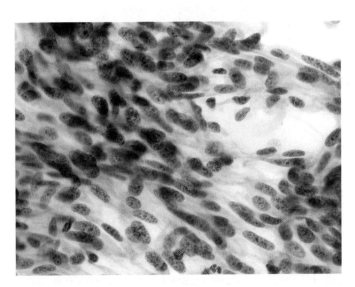

FIGURE 11.7. Undifferentiated (anaplastic) thyroid carcinoma. All neoplastic cells are strikingly spindle-shaped, resembling the cells of a sarcoma. Although chromatin is coarse, parachromatin clearing, prominent nucleoli, and nuclear irregularity are not apparent (smear, Papanicolaou stain).

In other cases, widespread tumor necrosis yields a sparsely cellular sample.[6] Due to rapid infiltrative tumor growth, aspirations can result in the acquisition of tumor cells admixed with extrathyroidal tissue such as skeletal muscle.

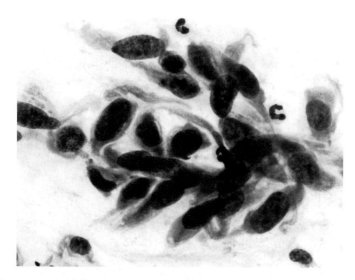

Figure 11.8. Undifferentiated (anaplastic) thyroid carcinoma. Tumor cells are notably spindle-shaped, with long, tapering cytoplasmic processes. Aside from nuclear enlargement, the atypia is relatively mild (smear, Diff-Quik stain).

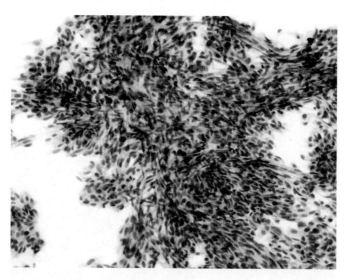

Figure 11.9. Undifferentiated (anaplastic) thyroid carcinoma. Tumors with a predominantly spindle-cell morphology can appear as microbiopsy fragments. A storiform pattern can be appreciated (smear, Papanicolaou stain).

Isolated cells and small to medium-sized cell groups can be found in most cases. In spindle-cell predominant UTCs, larger tumor fragments can reveal a storiform-like pattern.[5] Follicles, papillae, and trabecular/nested cell groups are not features of UTC.

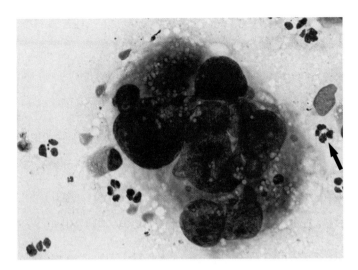

FIGURE 11.10. Undifferentiated (anaplastic) carcinoma. Bizarre multinucleated tumor giant cells may be found in some aspirations. The size of this tumor giant cell can be fully appreciated when compared to the adjacent neutrophils and malignant mononuclear cells (arrow) (smear, Diff-Quik).

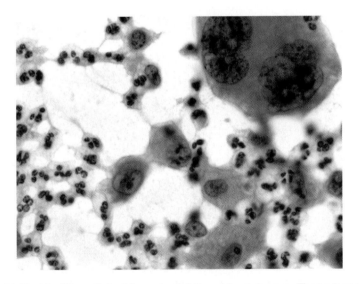

FIGURE 11.11. Undifferentiated (anaplastic) thyroid carcinoma. These tumors can be associated with abundant inflammatory cells, typically neutrophils. A multinucleated tumor giant cell with bizarre nuclear features and smaller, isolated, less anaplastic malignant cells are readily identifiable (smear, Papanicolaou stain).

Small to gigantic malignant cells may be epithelioid (round to polygonal) or spindle-shaped.[6,9,10] A given tumor often displays a mixture of cell shapes and sizes. Nuclear pleomorphism can be striking, with giant, bizarre,

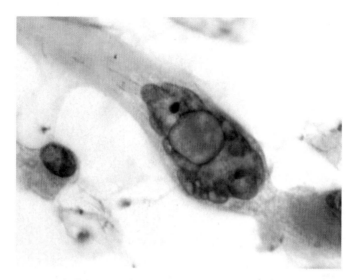

Figure 11.12. Undifferentiated (anaplastic) thyroid carcinoma. A giant spindle-shaped tumor cell has a massive intranuclear cytoplasmic pseudoinclusion. Other nuclear features include enlargement, contour irregularity, and a prominent nucleolus (smear, Papanicolaou stain).

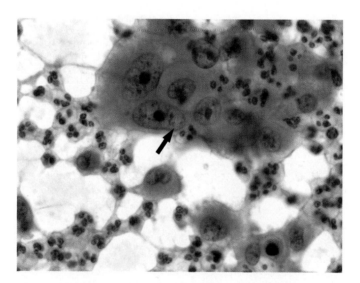

Figure 11.13. Undifferentiated (anaplastic) thyroid carcinoma. Epithelioid tumor cells display size variation, mononucleated and binucleated forms, macronucleoli, and clumped chromatin with parachromatin clearing (arrow). Acute inflammatory cells are present in the background (smear, Papanicolaou stain).

hyperchromatic forms.[6,9,10] Nuclei may be variably positioned within cells, but can be uniformly eccentric, resulting in a plasmacytoid morphology.[6] Intranuclear cytoplasmic pseudoinclusions, prominent nucleoli, clumped

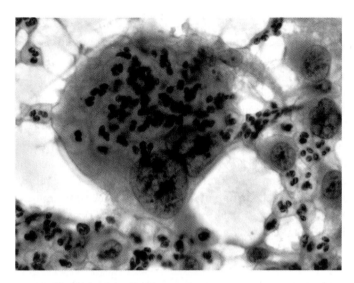

Figure 11.14. Undifferentiated (anaplastic) thyroid carcinoma. A multinucleated tumor giant cell demonstrates conspicuous intracytoplasmic neutrophilic infiltration (smear, Papanicolaou stain).

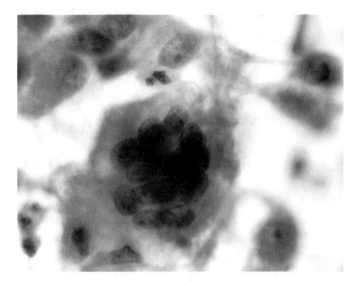

Figure 11.15. Undifferentiated (anaplastic) thyroid carcinoma. Some UTCs contain numerous non-neoplastic, osteoclast-like giant cells (center). Malignant cells are present in the background (smear, Papanicolaou stain).

chromatin, and parachromatin clearing may be identified.[6,9,10] Neutrophilic infiltration of tumor cells, osteoclast-like giant cells, necrosis, fibrotic tissue fragments and mitotic figures may be present in variable proportions.[6–10]

Some UTCs have a focus of co-existing well-differentiated and/or poorly differentiated thyroid carcinoma, most often papillary thyroid carcinoma,[4,5,8–10] but sometimes follicular carcinoma,[4,5,11] Hürthle cell carcinoma,[4,5] insular carcinoma[3,9] and other types of poorly differentiated carcinomas, or medullary thyroid carcinoma.[11] Consequently, it is feasible that several components can be observed in an aspiration specimen. Hence, thorough sampling and attention to the possibility of multiple components are imperative so that the identification of the most significant (i.e., least differentiated) cellular pattern is made. The frequent co-existence of a nidus of well differentiated thyroid cancers within a UTC suggests that UTC represents dedifferentiation of a well differentiated thyroid cancer through a multistep process of carcinogenesis.[1,11] This is supported by the occasional observation of UTC in metastatic foci from patients whose primary thyroid carcinomas were well differentiated.[4,11]

The most reliably positive immunostain in UTCs is pan-keratin, but rates of expression range from 50% to 100%.[5,12] Vimentin immunoexpression is also frequent.[5] Because thyroglobulin and TTF-1 are usually non-immunoreactive,[5,12] confusion can occur with sparsely cellular samples or aspirates of a spindled nature that are negative for keratin. In these cases, an erroneous diagnosis of sarcoma might be entertained, but primary sarcomas of the thyroid are very uncommon. Therefore tumor centered in the thyroid gland, based on imaging results, can help resolve this concern. Other entities in the differential diagnosis of UTC include insular carcinoma, medullary thyroid carcinoma, lymphoma and a metastasis. Compared to UTC, insular carcinoma has a lesser degree of nuclear atypia, a strikingly monotonous appearance, and a trabecular/nested architecture, and it lacks spindle-shaped cells and osteoclast-like giant cells. Medullary thyroid carcinoma, overall, is less pleomorphic than UTC and usually contains amyloid. Osteoclast-like giant cells and necrosis are absent in medullary carcinoma. If doubt remains after morphologic assessment, immmunochemistry can be helpful, in as much as medullary carcinomas are reactive for calcitonin and chromogranin, and UTCs are negative. Lymphoma can be excluded by the absence of lymphoglandular bodies and/or immunoreactivity for lymphoid markers. The most difficult mimic to exclude is often a metastasis (e.g., melanoma, sarcomatoid renal cell carcinoma, squamous cell or large cell carcinoma of the lung). Ruling out a metastasis requires knowledge of the patient's prior tumor history, clinical correlation (e.g., the size and the anatomic distribution of other extrathyroidal tumor masses), and targeted immunostaining.

In paucicellular aspirates due to necrosis and/or fibrosis, an underappreciation of rare malignant cells can lead to a misdiagnosis of a reactive process (e.g., Riedel thyroiditis).[7]

Management

The overall survival of patients with UTC has not changed significantly in 20 years. One-fifth of patients require tracheostomy due to airway obstruction during the course of their disease.[13]

Suppression with radioactive iodine is largely ineffective for the treatment of UTC.[4,13] Consequently, complete surgical resection, with or without pre-operative hyperfractionated radiotherapy and/or chemotherapy to enhance resectability through tumor shrinkage, is the optimal treatment strategy.[4,13] In cases where potential cure cannot be achieved, reducing the tumor burden through surgery facilitates the efficacy of post-operative radiation and/or chemotherapy.[13] In patients fit enough to employ these regimens, length of survival is improved.[5,13] Not surprisingly, younger patients (<45 years old) and individuals with smaller tumors without extensive extrathyroidal tissue invasion or metastases have the best outcome.[2,4,5]

Squamous Cell Carcinoma of the Thyroid

Squamous cell carcinoma (SQC) of the thyroid accounts for 1% or less of thyroid cancers. Like UTC, it occurs in the elderly and has a similar (dismal) prognosis.

Definition

Squamous cell carcinoma of the thyroid is a malignant tumor that shows exclusively squamous differentiation.

Criteria (Fig. 11.16)

Cytologic samples are composed almost exclusively of large, pleomorphic keratinized cells.

Necrosis may be present.

Explanatory Notes and Management

Most squamous cell carcinomas of the thyroid are poorly differentiated. The differential diagnosis includes UTC and metastatic SQC. Primary squamous cell carcinomas of the thyroid are morphologically and immunochemically indistinguishable from squamous cell carcinomas of other organs. For this reason, correlation with clinical and imaging findings is essential for excluding a metastasis. Clinical management of squamous cell carcinomas of the thyroid is the same as for UTC.

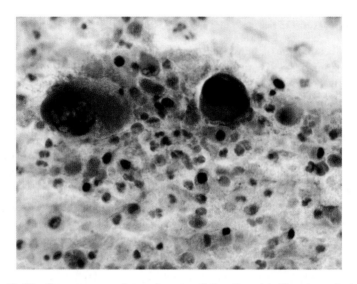

Figure 11.16. Squamous cell carcinoma of the thyroid. The sample is composed of large pleomorphic cells with conspicuous dense orangeophilia of the cytoplasm. There is abundant necrosis, and nuclei show degenerative changes (i.e., dark, smudged and/or marginated chromatin) (smear, Papanicolaou stain).

Sample Reports

The general category "MALIGNANT" is used whenever the cytomorphologic features are conclusive for malignancy. If an aspirate is interpreted as malignant, it is implied that the sample is adequate for evaluation. An explicit statement of adequacy is optional. Descriptive comments that follow are used to sub-classify the malignancy and summarize the results of special studies, if any. If the findings are suspicious but not conclusive for malignancy, the general category "Suspicious for malignancy" should be used (see Chap. 7).

Example 1:
MALIGNANT.
Undifferentiated (anaplastic) thyroid carcinoma.
  Note: Immunohistochemistry performed on cell block preparations shows
    that the malignant cells are focally immunoreactive for pan-cytokeratin
    AE1/3 and are negative for thyroglobulin and TTF-1.

Example 2:
  MALIGNANT.
  Poorly differentiated carcinoma, consistent with undifferentiated (anaplastic)
    thyroid carcinoma.

Note: Immunocytochemistry performed on cytocentrifuge preparations shows that the malignant cells are focally immunoreactive for cytokeratins AE1/3 and vimentin, and are negative for thyroglobulin, TTF-1, HMB-45, and S-100 protein. The prior clinical history of malignant melanoma is noted.

Example 3:

MALIGNANT.

Consistent with squamous cell carcinoma of the thyroid.

Note: The distinction between a primary squamous cell carcinoma of the thyroid and a metastasis to the thyroid from a primary elsewhere is not possible by cytomorphology or immunochemistry. Correlation with clinical and imaging findings is advised.

References

1. Agarwal S, Rao RS, Parikh DM, et al. Histologic trends in thyroid cancer 1969–1993: a clinico-pathologic analysis of the relative proportion of anaplastic carcinoma of the thyroid. *J Surg Oncol.* 1996;63(4):251-255.
2. Hundahl SA, Fleming ID, Fremgen AM, et al. A National Cancer Data Base report on 53,856 cases of thyroid carcinoma treated in the U.S., 1985–1995. *Cancer* 1998;83(12): 2638-2648.
3. Lam KY, Lo CY, Chan KW, et al. Insular and anaplastic carcinoma of the thyroid: a 45-year comparative study at a single institution and a review of the significance of p53 and p21. *Ann Surg.* 2000;231(3):329-338.
4. Aldinger KA, Samaan NA, Ibanez M, et al. Anaplastic carcinoma of the thyroid: a review of 84 cases of spindle and giant cell carcinoma of the thyroid. *Cancer.* 1978;41(6):2267-2275.
5. Venkatesh YS, Ordonez NG, Schultz PN, et al. Anaplastic carcinoma of the thyroid. A clinicopathologic study of 121 cases. *Cancer* 1990;66(2):321-330.
6. Us-Krasovec M, Golouh R, Auersperg M, et al. Anaplastic thyroid carcinoma in fine needle aspirates. *Acta Cytol.* 1996;40(5):953-958.
7. Deshpande AH, Munshi MM, Bobhate SK. Cytological diagnosis of paucicellular variant of anaplastic carcinoma of thyroid: report of two cases. *Cytopathology.* 2001;12(3):203-208.
8. Carcangiu ML, Steeper T, Zampi G, Rosai J, Anaplastic thyroid carcinoma. A study of 70 cases. *Am J Clin Pathol* 1985;83(2):135-158.
9. Brooke PK, Hameed M, Zakowski MF. Fine-needle aspiration of anaplastic thyroid carcinoma with varied cytologic and histologic patterns: a case report. *Diagn Cytopathol.* 1994;11(1):60-63.
10. Guarda LA, Peterson CE, Hall W, et al. Anaplastic thyroid carcinoma: cytomorphology and clinical implications of fine-needle aspiration. *Diagn Cytopathol.* 1991;7(1):63-67.
11. Oktay MH, Smolkin MB, Williams M, et al. Metastatic anaplastic carcinoma of the thyroid mimicking squamous cell carcinoma: report of a case of a challenging cytologic diagnosis. *Acta Cytol.* 2006;50(2):201-204.
12. Miettinen M, Franssila KO. Variable expression of keratins and nearly uniform lack of thyroid transcription factor 1 in thyroid anaplastic carcinoma. *Hum Pathol.* 2000;31(9):1139-1145.
13. Lang BH, Lo CY. Surgical options in undifferentiated thyroid carcinoma. *World J Surg.* 2007;31(5):969-977.

Chapter 12

Metastatic Tumors and Lymphomas

Lester J. Layfield, Jerry Waisman, and Kristen A. Atkins

Background

Metastases from distant organs and direct extension of tumors from adjacent structures are uncommon but important to recognize in fine needle aspiration (FNA) samples of thyroid nodules. In rare cases, a metastasis to the thyroid can even be the initial presentation of a distant malignancy. Tumors of nearby structures that can involve the thyroid include those of the pharynx, larynx, esophagus, mediastinum, and nearby lymph nodes.[1] The most common origins of metastases to the thyroid are cancers of the lung, breast, skin (especially melanoma), colon, and kidney.[2–6] The incidence varies in surgical vs. autopsy series (2.7–4.0%). Metastases, including micrometastases, are found in up to 10% of cancer necropsies.[2] Metastatic carcinomas characteristically present in one of three patterns; (1) multiple small discrete nodules (less than 2 mm); (2) solitary large nodules; and (3) diffuse involvement. When small nodules are present, neoplastic cells are admixed with indigenous follicular epithelial cells. With large nodules, the malignant cells are not mixed with follicular epithelial cells. With routine and special stains, distinction of metastatic carcinoma from a primary neoplasm of the thyroid is achievable, but, to assist with this, clinicians are expected to supply the history of malignancy on the requisition form.[7]

Malignant lymphomas can arise in the thyroid as primary malignancies or involve the thyroid gland secondarily as part of systemic disease.[8] Most primary thyroid lymphomas are of B-cell type.[8] Lymphomas represent approximately 5% of thyroid neoplasms, usually associated with Hashimoto thyroiditis.[8] Plasma cell tumors and Hodgkin lymphoma are rare in the thyroid gland.

Syed Z. Ali and Edmund S. Cibas (eds.), *The Bethesda System for Reporting Thyroid Cytopathology*, DOI 10.1007/ 978-0-387-87666-5_12, © Springer Science+Business Media, LLC 2010

Metastatic Renal Cell Carcinoma

A majority of the metastatic renal cell carcinomas (RCC) are of the clear cell type and present as solitary or multiple nodules,[9,10] occurring as long as 20 years following the resection of the primary neoplasm.[10]

Definition

Metastatic RCC is a malignant neoplasm arising from one of the kidneys and involving the thyroid gland.

Criteria (Figs. 12.1 and 12.2)

Samples show moderate to high cellularity.

Cells are dispersed individually and in small clusters, fragmented papillae, or sheets.

Cells have abundant pale, finely granular, clear or vacuolated cytoplasm.

Nuclei are round to oval, often with large nucleoli.

Samples are often bloody.

Explanatory Notes

Metastatic RCC displays moderately to highly cellular, often bloody, preparations.[11] Cells appear singly and in cohesive clusters, fragmented papillae, and sheets (Fig. 12.1). The individual cells have abundant pale and finely

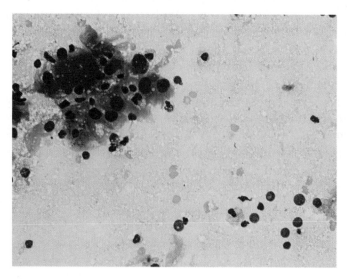

FIGURE 12.1. Metastatic renal cell carcinoma, clear cell type. The malignant cells have abundant granular and vacuolated cytoplasm (smear, Diff-Quik stain).

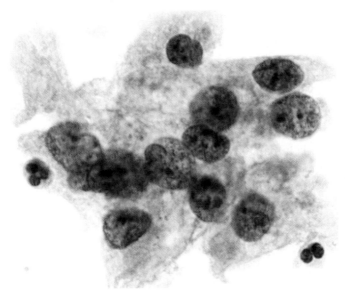

FIGURE 12.2. Metastatic renal carcinoma, clear cell type. Cells in a small cluster have abundant finely vacuolated cytoplasm (ThinPrep, Papanicolaou stain).

vacuolated cytoplasm with Romanowsky-stained preparations or clear when a Papanicolaou stain is used (Fig. 12.2). The nuclear/cytoplasmic ratio is low. The nuclei are round or oval and vary in size and shape. The nuclear chromatin is finely granular. The prominence of the nucleoli is directly proportional to the grade of the RCC. Intranuclear cytoplasmic pseudoinclusions are found in a minority of metastatic RCC. A characteristic of high grade RCC in air-dried smears is strands of pink, hyaline, or fibrillary stroma with attached fusiform cells.

The distinction between clear cell RCC and follicular and Hürthle cell neoplasms is difficult, particularly if the RCC is occult, or if the history of RCC is not provided on the requisition form.[12] Immunostaining for thyroid markers (e.g., thyroglobulin, thyroid transcription factor 1 (TTF1), and calcitonin), and RCC markers (e.g., RCC antigen, CD10) can aid in the differential diagnosis.

Metastatic Malignant Melanoma

Definition

Metastatic malignant melanoma (MM) is a malignancy derived from or differentiating towards melanocytes that arises from skin or, less commonly, extra-cutaneous sites and involves the thyroid gland.

Criteria (Figs. 12.3 and 12.4)

Samples are moderately or markedly cellular and most cells are noncohesive.

Cells are variable in size and shape and include plasmacytoid, spindle-shaped, and anaplastic forms.

Nuclei are large and often eccentrically placed.

Intranuclear cytoplasmic pseudoinclusions can be present.

Intracytoplasmic pigment is not common but can be seen as fine granules in neoplastic cells or coarse granules in histiocytes.

Cells are usually immunoreactive for S-100 protein, melanA, and HMB45.

Explanatory Notes

Aspirates from metastatic MM are characterized by many dispersed cells, with marked variability in size and oval, plasmacytoid, fusiform, and anaplastic forms (Fig. 12.3).[13] Eccentrically positioned nuclei are usually round or ovoid and vary in size and number. The cells typically have well defined cytoplasm. Intranuclear cytoplasmic pseudoinclusions are seen. Intracytoplasmic pigment is not common but may be seen as fine granules in the cytoplasm or dark staining in perinuclear areas. More often, melanin is found as coarse granules in histiocytes (Fig. 12.4).[13]

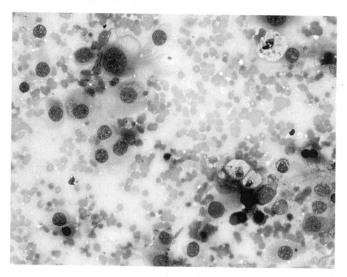

FIGURE 12.3. Metastatic melanoma. The malignant cells are isolated and loosely aggregated. They are large, oval and plasmacytoid cells with abundant granular cytoplasm, hyperchromatic nuclei, and prominent nucleoli. Foamy histiocytes are present (smear, Diff-Quik stain).

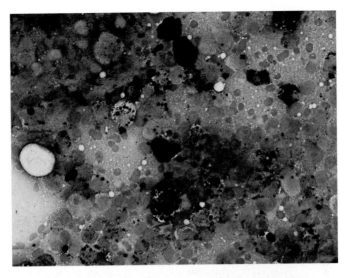

FIGURE 12.4. Metastatic melanoma. Most of the pigment is engulfed by macrophages ("melanophages") (smear, Diff-Quik stain).

At times, separation of MM from undifferentiated (anaplastic) thyroid carcinoma (UTC) is difficult. Smears obtained from MM are generally more cellular than those of UTC, with more intact isolated cells. Immunostains can be helpful: MM is positive for S-100 protein, HMB45, and melanA; these markers are negative in UTC.

Metastatic Adenocarcinoma from the Breast

Definition

Metastatic adenocarcinoma of the breast is an epithelial malignancy arising from or differentiating towards mammary epithelium and involving the thyroid gland.

Criteria (Fig. 12.5)

Samples are of moderate to high cellularity with a uniform population of oval or polygonal cells.

Cells lie singly and in small clusters; the isolated cells retain their cytoplasm.

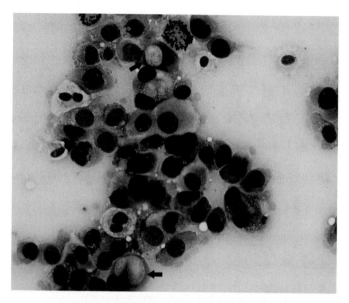

Figure 12.5. Metastatic ductal carcinoma of the breast. Medium-sized cells with large eccentric nuclei and intracytoplasmic vacuolar purple granules (magenta bodies, *arrows*) (smear, Diff-Quik stain).

Cells are often immunoreactive for estrogen and progesterone receptors and negative for TTF-1 and thyroglobulin.

Explanatory Notes

Metastases from adenocarcinoma of the breast are one of the most common of the metastatic lesions to the thyroid gland,[14] and most are infiltrating ductal carcinomas. Smears are of moderate to high cellularity with a uniform population of polygonal or oval cells. The cells appear singly and in clusters, and single cells retain the cytoplasm. The clusters are angular.

On air-dried smears, purple cytoplasmic inclusions (magenta bodies) may be seen in metastatic breast carcinoma of both ductal and lobular types (Fig. 12.5). Many metastatic adenocarcinomas of the breast have cells similar to neoplastic follicular cells. The cells of infiltrating ductal adenocarcinoma are larger than those of follicular neoplasms but smaller than those seen in primary Hürthle cell neoplasms. The presence of microfollicles favors a thyroid neoplasm over metastatic mammary carcinoma.

Immunohistochemical stains for thyroid-specific antigens (e.g., thyroglobulin, TTF1, and calcitonin) and breast-specific markers (e.g., estrogen and progesterone receptors) can be helpful for the separation of metastatic mammary carcinoma from benign and neoplastic thyroid follicular cells.

Metastatic Pulmonary Carcinoma

The appearance of smears from bronchogenic carcinomas depends on the primary tumor. Metastatic small cell carcinoma (SmCC) may resemble insular thyroid carcinoma, but has more fragile nuclei and cytoplasm and thus greater smearing artifact than found with primary thyroid neoplasms. Both metastatic pulmonary SmCC and insular carcinoma may be immunoreactive for neuron-specific enolase (NSE), chromogranin, and synaptophysin, whereas only insular carcinomas are thyroglobulin-positive.

Adenocarcinomas of pulmonary origin are composed of medium-sized to large cells lying in sheets or clusters/balls (Figs. 12.6 and 12.7). The cells may be columnar with round to oval eccentric nuclei and prominent nucleoli. Both, primary thyroid tumors and non-small cell bronchogenic carcinomas are TTF1-positive, precluding this as a distinguishing marker. Bronchogenic adenocarcinomas are characteristically of higher nuclear grade than follicular neoplasms of the thyroid gland. Metastatic carcinomas of pulmonary origin are more likely to contain intracytoplasmic mucin and show squamous differentiation.

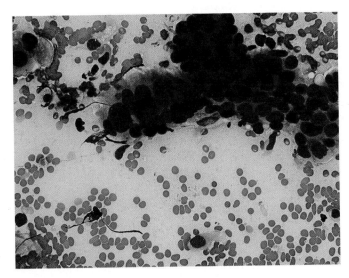

Figure 12.6. Metastatic non-small cell lung carcinoma. Irregular cell clusters and spherical groups are composed of polygonal and columnar cells (smear, Diff-Quik stain).

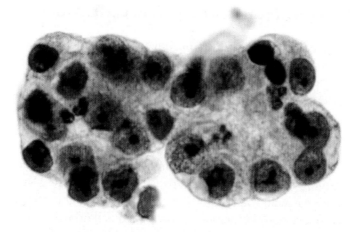

FIGURE 12.7. Metastatic non-small cell lung carcinoma. Medium-sized cells have large nuclei and prominent nucleoli. The cells are arranged in spherical clusters (ThinPrep, Papanicolaou stain).

Other Metastatic Malignancies

Examples of less common metastatic neoplasms to the thyroid gland are shown in Figs. 12.8–12.10. Diagnosis by FNA is contingent upon the clinical history, often with the support of immunohistochemical staining.

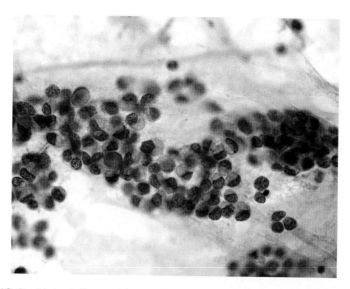

FIGURE 12.8. Metastatic gastric signet-ring cell carcinoma. Uniform dispersed cells have a high N/C ratio and intracytoplasmic mucinous vacuoles (smear, Diff-Quik stain) (Photograph courtesy of Dr. QK Li, The Johns Hopkins Hospital, Baltimore, MD.).

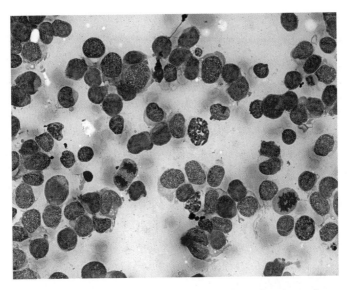

FIGURE **12.9.** Metastatic Merkel cell carcinoma. Dispersed small, round, blue cells have a high N/C ratio and frequent mitotic figures (smear, Diff-Quik stain).

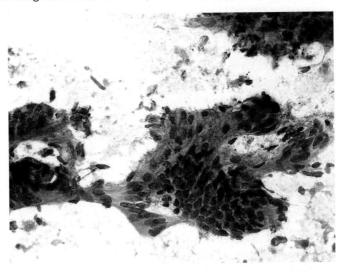

FIGURE **12.10.** Metastatic colonic adenocarcinoma. Columnar cells with nuclear stratification are associated with granular necrotic debris in the background (smear, Papanicolaou stain).

Lymphoma Involving the Thyroid Gland

Definition

Hodgkin and non-Hodgkin lymphomas are malignancies of lymphoid cells, most commonly B-cells, and arise in the thyroid gland as a primary malignancy or involve the thyroid gland secondarily.

Criteria

Samples are often markedly cellular and composed of noncohesive round to slightly oval cells.

The background contains numerous lymphoglandular bodies, best seen with a Romanowsky-type stain on air-dried preparations.

Cells of marginal zone lymphoma are about twice the size of a small mature lymphocyte.

Nuclei have vesicular ("open") chromatin (with Papanicolaou-stained preparations) and small nucleoli.

Diffuse large B-cell lymphomas (DLBL) contain cells with moderate to abundant basophilic cytoplasm on air-dried preparations stained with a Romanowsky-type stain.

Nuclei have coarse chromatin with one or more prominent nucleoli.

Explanatory Notes

The majority of lymphomas arising within the thyroid gland are non-Hodgkin lymphomas (NHL) of B-cell phenotype (98%),[15] and two-thirds are preceded by Hashimoto thyroiditis. Most NHLs of the thyroid gland are either DLBL or extranodal marginal zone B-cell lymphomas of mucosa-associated lymphoid tissue (MALT). Distinction of thyroid lymphoma from Hashimoto thyroiditis may be difficult.[16] There are at least three different patterns of lymphoma on FNA.[17] One is characterized by mixture of small and large lymphocytes. This pattern can be seen in Hashimoto thyroiditis as well, but the absence of oncocytes, follicular epithelial cells, and plasma cells favors lymphoma. The second pattern is characterized by a monotonous population of large lymphoid cells and is morphologically diagnostic of lymphoma. The third pattern is characterized by a monomorphous population of small lymphocytes, which may represent lymphoma or inactive thyroiditis. Immunophenotyping studies are essential for the diagnosis of lymphoma in morphologically equivocal cases. A clonal relationship between Hashimoto thyroiditis and thyroid lymphoma may exist,[18] and clonal B-cell populations by flow cytometry have been reported in patients with Hashimoto thyroiditis.[19,20] Caution is advised, therefore, in interpreting results.

Secondary involvement of the thyroid gland by lymphoma is more frequent than primary disease. Approximately 20% of patients with disseminated lymphoma demonstrate thyroid involvement.

Extranodal Marginal Zone B-Cell Lymphoma (MALT Lymphoma)

FNA preparations from MALT lymphomas are markedly cellular and composed of lymphoid cells in isolation and in clusters.[21,22] Numerous lymphoglandular bodies are present. The cells are small to intermediate-sized, about twice as large as a small mature lymphocyte.[21] Most cells have a moderate amount of cytoplasm surrounding slightly vesicular nuclei with "open" (i.e., pale) chromatin (Fig. 12.11). Small nucleoli are present. A small number of larger cells are present with eccentric nuclei, coarse chromatin, and prominent nucleoli. These cells are admixed with lesser numbers of centrocytic cells, monocytoid B-cells, and plasma cells. In some cases, plasmacytoid cells dominate.[23] Often, a small number of follicular and oncocytic thyroid epithelial cells are admixed with the lymphoid cells.[21]

Diffuse Large B-Cell Lymphoma

Smears of DLBL are highly cellular with many lymphoglandular bodies in the background. The smears are monotonous, composed of noncohesive

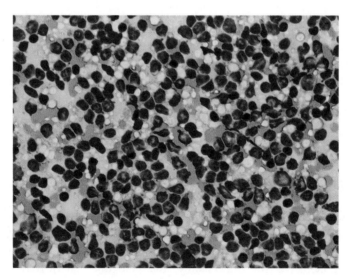

FIGURE 12.11. Primary MALT-type lymphoma of the thyroid. There is an abundance of uniform intermediate-sized cells with small nucleoli and granular chromatin (smear, Diff-Quik stain).

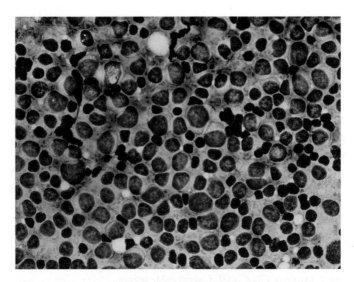

Figure 12.12. Diffuse large B-cell lymphoma of the thyroid. The smear is cellular and composed mostly of large lymphoid cells whose nuclei are three to five times larger than those of the smaller lymphocytes (smear, Diff-Quik stain).

large lymphoid cells (Fig. 12.12).[21] With air-dried smears stained with a Romanowsky-type stain, the cells have moderate to abundant basophilic cytoplasm. The nuclei possess coarse chromatin with one or more prominent nucleoli.[21] Nuclei stripped of cytoplasm are numerous, and necrotic debris may be present. Flow cytometry reveals light chain monoclonality with CD45- and CD20-positive neoplastic cells.[24] Follicular cells are usually absent. Separation of these lymphomas from Hashimoto thyroiditis is straightforward.[24]

Sample Reports

The general category "MALIGNANT" is used whenever the clinical and microscopic features are conclusive. The type of metastatic or lymphoid malignancy should be stated whenever possible. If features are suspicious but not conclusive for malignancy, the category "SUSPICIOUS FOR MALIGNANCY" is used. Some aspirates, particularly those that raise the possibility of a lymphoma of MALT-type but lacking corroborative immunophenotyping data, are more appropriately categorized as "ATYPIA OF UNDETERMINED SIGNIFICANCE (AUS)" (See Chap. 4, Sample Report Example 9). If an aspirate is interpreted as Malignant, Suspicious, or AUS, it is implied that the sample is adequate for evaluation (An explicit statement of adequacy is optional).

Example 1:
> MALIGNANT.
> Diffuse large B-cell lymphoma.
> Note: Flow cytometry shows a CD45-, CD20-positive monoclonal B-cell population.

Example 2:
> SUSPICIOUS FOR MALIGNANCY.
> Suspicious for metastatic adenocarcinoma of the breast.

References

1. Willis RA. *The spread of tumors in the human body*. London: Butterworth; 1952: 271-275.
2. Disibio G, French SW. Metastatic patterns of cancers: results from a large autopsy study. *Arch Pathol Lab Med*. 2008;132(6):931-939.
3. Czech JM, Lichtor TR, Carney JA, van Heerden JA. Neoplasms metastatic to the thyroid gland. *Surg Gynecol Obstet*. 1982;155(4):503-505.
4. Ivy HK. Cancer metastatic to the thyroid: a diagnostic problem. *Mayo Clin Proc*. 1984;59(12):856-859.
5. Shimaoka K, Sokal JE, Pickren JW. Metastatic neoplasms in the thyroid gland. Pathological and clinical findings. *Cancer*. 1962;15:557-565.
6. Schroder S, Burk CG, de Heer K. Metastases of the thyroid gland–morphology and clinical aspects of 25 secondary thyroid neoplasms. *Langenbecks Arch Chir*. 1987;370(1):25-35.
7. Cibas ES, Alexander EK, Benson CB, et al. Indications for thyroid FNA and pre-FNA requirements: a synopsis of the National Cancer Institute Thyroid Fine Needle Aspiration State of the Science Conference. *Diagn Cytopathol*. 2008;36(6):390-399.
8. Derringer GA, Thompson LDR, Frommelt RA, Bijwaard KE, Heffess CS, Abbondanzo SL. Malignant lymphoma of the thyroid gland: a clinicopathologic study of 108 cases. *Am J Surg Pathol*. 2000;24:623-639.
9. Lehur PA, Cote RA, Poisson J, Boctor M, Elhilali M, Kandalaft N. Thyroid metastasis of clear-cell renal carcinoma. *Can Med Assoc J*. 1983;128(2):154-156.
10. Shima H, Mori H, Takahashi M, Nakamura S, Miura K, Tarao M. A case of renal cell carcinoma solitarily metastasized to thyroid 20 years after the resection of primary tumor. *Pathol Res Pract*. 1985;179(6):666-672.
11. Lasser A, Rothman JG, Calamia VJ. Renal-cell carcinoma metastatic to the thyroid. Aspiration cytology and histologic findings. *Acta Cytol*. 1985;29(5):856-858.
12. Variakojis D, Getz ML, Paloyan E, Straus FH. Papillary clear cell carcinoma of the thyroid gland. *Hum Pathol*. 1975;6(3):384-390.
13. Layfield LJ, Ostrzega N. Fine needle aspirate smear morphology in metastatic melanoma. *Acta Cytol*. 1989;33(5):606-612.
14. Smith SA, Gharib H, Goellner JR. Fine-needle aspiration: usefulness for diagnosis and management of metastatic carcinoma to the thyroid. *Arch Intern Med*. 1987;147: 311-312.
15. Pedersen RK, Pedersen NT. Primary non-Hodgkin's lymphoma of the thyroid gland: a population based study. *Histopathology*. 1996;28(1):25-32.
16. Lerma E, Arguelles R, Rigla M, et al. Comparative findings of lymphocytic thyroiditis and thyroid lymphoma. *Acta Cytol*. 2003;47(4):575-580.

17. Kossev P, Livolsi V. Lymphoid lesions of the thyroid: review in light of the revised European-American lymphoma classification and upcoming World Health Organization classification. *Thyroid.* 1999;9(12):1273-1280.
18. Moshynska OV, Saxena A. Clonal relationship between Hashimoto thyroiditis and thyroid lymphoma. *J Clin Pathol.* 2008;61(4):438-444.
19. Saxena A, Alport EC, Moshynska O, Kanthan R, Boctor MA. Clonal B cell populations in a minority of patients with Hashimoto's thyroiditis. *J Clin Pathol.* 2004;57(12): 1258-1263.
20. Chen HI, Akpolat I, Mody DR, et al. Restricted kappa/lambda light chain ratio by flow cytometry in germinal center B cells in Hashimoto thyroiditis. *Am J Clin Pathol.* 2006;125(1):42-48.
21. Sangalli G, Serio G, Zampatti C, Lomuscio G, Colombo L. Fine needle aspiration cytology of primary lymphoma of the thyroid: a report of 17 cases. *Cytopathology.* 2001;12(4): 257-263.
22. Murphy BA, Meda BA, Buss DH, Geisinger KR. Marginal zone and mantle cell lymphomas: assessment of cytomorphology in subtyping small B-cell lymphomas. *Diagn Cytopathol.* 2003;28(3):126-130.
23. Al-Marzooq YM, Chopra R, Younis M, Al-Mulhim AS, Al-Mommatten MI, Al-Omran SH. Thyroid low-grade B-cell lymphoma (MALT type) with extreme plasmacytic differentiation: report of a case diagnosed by fine-needle aspiration and flow cytometric study. *Diagn Cytopathol.* 2004;31(1):52-56.
24. Tani E, Skoog L. Fine needle aspiration cytology and immunocytochemistry in the diagnosis of lymphoid lesions of the thyroid gland. *Acta Cytol.* 1989;33(1):48-52.

Index

Sec p 59